NO MORE NORMAL

Also by Alastair Santhouse

Head First: A Psychiatrist's Stories of Mind and Body

Dr Alastair Santhouse

No More Normal

Mental Health in an Age of Over-Diagnosis

GRANTA

Granta Publications, 12 Addison Avenue, London W11 4QR
First published in Great Britain by Granta Books, 2025

Neither the publisher nor the author is engaged in rendering
professional advice or services to the individual reader. The ideas, procedures
and suggestions contained in this book are not intended as a substitute for
consulting with your physician. All matters regarding your health require
medical supervision. Neither the author nor the publisher shall be liable
or responsible for any loss or damage allegedly arising from any
information or suggestion in this book.

The stories chronicled in this book are based on many years of practice.
However, maintaining patient confidentiality is of utmost importance and
so the author has taken care to remove any identifying clinical or personal
information. Patient names have been chosen at random. Some of the
case studies are an amalgam of several patients.

A CIP catalogue record for this book is available from the British Library.

1 3 5 7 9 10 8 6 4 2

ISBN 978 1 80351 114 6 (hardback)
ISBN 978 1 80351 116 0 (ebook)

Typeset in Bembo by Iram Allam
Printed and bound by CPI Group (UK) Ltd, Croydon, CR0 4YY
www.granta.com

MIX
Paper | Supporting
responsible forestry
FSC
www.fsc.org   FSC® C171272

To my parents, Carl and Arleen Santhouse

Contents

1

Introduction

Psychiatry, the area of medicine I have specialised in for over a quarter of a century, is at a crossroads. What counts as a diagnosis and what counts as normal mental health are becoming more flexible. Increasingly, the concept of normal is not decided by evidence, or even by psychiatrists, but by social trends and appeals to emotion. Burgeoning theories and treatments, expectations of good mental health and contentment, and the language of wellness have all created a climate that has influenced how mental health and illness are thought about and experienced.

Many of these changes have been driven by the highest motives and have had positive effects. Each generation wants to improve on what has gone before. The stigma that had for so long added to the distress of people suffering from mental health conditions has been removed or lessened, and more people now feel willing to come forward to access treatment. We value virtues such as compassion and kindness as the foundation for a progressive society, and they are undoubtedly important. Yet such emphasis has started to lead us to explain the cares of life, of suffering and difference, within the framework of illness.

These changes have been significant. To demonstrate empathy, we are now medicalising people who in previous generations would have been considered normal. By telling people they have a right to enjoy perfect mental harmony, and if they do not, this is due to underlying factors beyond their control, we prevent people from experiencing the personal growth that difficulty, adversity and hard truths bring.

A great deal of medicine is about trying to interpret a subjective, internal and individual experience. This can be hard enough to measure in physical medicine, even when there is an obvious visible or detectable bodily cause, but the challenge is even greater in psychiatry. Our diagnoses rely not on the results of physical investigations but on the consensus of a body of experts, all of whom carry their own interpretations of the research findings and comparisons with what is normal health. This may be seen in how we consider, for example, what is a normal reaction to loss and bereavement, or whether or not we consider psychiatry even has any place in these areas. Of all the medical specialisms, psychiatry is the most sensitive to social and cultural values, which have a bearing on how we all conceive of and talk about our experiences.

As a clinician, I frequently ask myself whether all the changes we have made in our understanding of what is normal represent progress. Are we moving in a linear way to an ever more enlightened goal of human understanding? Or are we caught in a circular process in which fashions and dogma will forever bring us back to the beginning, with no genuine concept of normal mental health, just endlessly changing beliefs and values?

'Normal' is a crucial concept in psychiatry; all mental illness is defined by it. This makes sense. There needs to be a yardstick against which we measure an individual's mental health. But if normal is so changeable, how can we rely on our judgement about what counts as abnormal? How much suspicion do you need before being considered paranoid? How often must you check something before being investigated for obsessive compulsive disorder (OCD)? How sad can someone be after a bereavement before it becomes depression? Where does unrequited love end and mental illness begin? What events count as traumatic? Who gets to decide, and how do they reach their decisions?

One study that caught my attention was a survey conducted by the National Union of Students in 2015. It was reported[1,2] that 78% of students had experienced a mental health problem in the past year. As Professor Sir Simon Wessely, former president of the Royal College of Psychiatrists, commented in the *British Medical Journal* (*BMJ*),[3] 'One wonders what's happening when you have 78% of students telling their union they have mental health problems – you have to think, "Well, this seems unlikely."'

I don't doubt that being a student can involve some difficult moments. I remember from my own student days the relentless volume of work, the intensity of exams, social pressures – and as for relationships, my status as single was such a constant feature of my university life that I began to wonder if something was wrong with me. To this are now added student loan debt, the prevalence of social media and the impact of technology on the job market. All of these are life's difficulties and stresses to be navigated. The novelty is in framing these difficulties as mental health problems. The students in the survey did not see themselves as unhappy or distressed, but rather as ill.

It is self-evident that if the boundary of where normal mental health lies is constantly changing, then what counts as a diagnosable mental or neurodevelopmental disorder must be changing too. And changing it is. As the criteria for being diagnosed with autism spectrum disorder (ASD), for example, are being loosened, they start to encompass many people who would have previously had no reason for contact with mental health services. This includes those who are socially awkward or idiosyncratic but broadly functioning in society, with careers and relationships. Rates of ASD have increased sharply, by 787% between 1998 and 2018 according to one large study.[4] In former times, to be diagnosed with autism meant that severe disabilities in communication and learning were evident. Those individuals diagnosed usually attended special schools and were frequently non-verbal. This is no longer the case, and we are now diagnosing people with far milder symptoms, which means not only that more people are being diagnosed than ever before, but also that people with more severe difficulties are finding it harder to access services. It can also lead to problems with research trials for ASD treatments. If the population being tested includes some people with only mild symptoms, say a lack of social awareness or poor social communication, how do we know they have the same diagnosis as those with severe learning difficulties who are entirely non-verbal? In such cases, defining normal is not just an abstract matter of interest; it is a fundamental value in deciding who gets care and who does not, and who can re-evaluate their life difficulties as because of their diagnosis, rather than owing to factors relating to their personality, phase of life, or circumstances.

In the decades since I qualified in 1992, I have worked on the frontline of psychiatry, including nearly twenty years as a psychiatrist in a central London general hospital. Over that time, I have seen the immense consequences for an individual of the label of mental illness. It affects an individual's self-perception, it removes the feeling of control that someone may have over their own life and destiny, and it can introduce feelings of helplessness in the face of life's challenges. These challenges – suffering, unhappiness, anger, indignation, resentment, suspicion, infatuation, disinterest in sex, jealousy, elation – have been normal human emotions since the beginning of time. To think of them otherwise is to misunderstand people altogether and can lead to unnecessary treatments for diagnoses that aren't justified.

Why then are we moving towards an ever-expanding lexicon of psychiatric diagnoses? The *Diagnostic and Statistical Manual of Mental Disorders* (DSM), the reference point for all psychiatric diagnoses, shows that the number of diagnoses you can suffer from has increased more than fourfold in the past seventy years.[5] Yet are we really less psychologically healthy than previous generations? As we will see, a current trend in society means that if someone says they have a mental disorder, they will invariably find someone to endorse that label. I see this increasingly in my clinics – the pathologising of normal emotions, of 'trauma-informed' diagnostic formulations and ever-expanding types of therapy. Even the notion of 'normal' itself is sometimes seen as controversial and discriminatory. On the positive side, we now live in a society less ready to stigmatise and marginalise people who do not conform to a narrow set of norms. In a way unimaginable to previous generations, people are proud to own a diagnostic label, sometimes to the extent that the socially understood meaning of the label is also changing. In some cases, a label has come to feel less like a psychiatric diagnosis and more like a facet of a person's social identity. On the flip side, the number of people who enjoy or perhaps perceive that they enjoy – normal mental health is getting progressively lower.

The Health Foundation produced a report[6] that highlighted the extent of the economic and workforce impact of poorer mental health. Mental ill health is now the commonest cause of work-limiting conditions for those aged forty-four and under. This eclipses musculoskeletal and chronic health conditions, which have traditionally been the main work-limiting conditions. The report goes on to say: 'More than four times as many young workers report that their mental health affects the type or amount of work they can do, than was the case only a decade ago.'

One explanation for the figures is that they really are what they seem to be, namely that mental illness rates have soared for reasons we don't fully understand, and that young people are now being disproportionately affected. The report itself speculates that maybe more people are prepared to come forward now, with the successful campaign to reduce the stigma of mental illness. Maybe that's true, but it would not explain everything, and particularly why people who could work before are unable to do so now. Another, perhaps more likely, explanation is that at the milder end of the spectrum, more problems are being reclassified as mental health diagnoses, and more people are willing to frame their problems in medical terms.

The last decade or so has seen a change in our use of terms in describing psychological distress. Increasingly there has been a conflation of the terms 'mental illness' and 'mental health'. They seem to mean different things to different people. Does mental health mean the absence of mental illness? Or is it about a fully self-actualised state of mental harmony, a state of perfect mental equilibrium? When someone says that their mental health has been affected by an event, what are they communicating? Have they become mentally ill, or are they distressed but not 'ill' in any normal sense?

The World Health Organization has a definition that, to my mind, reflects this confusion. It says in a fact sheet[7] that 'Mental health is more than the absence of mental disorders. It exists on a complex continuum, which is experienced differently from one person to the next, with varying degrees of difficulty and distress and potentially very different social and clinical outcomes.' It goes on to say that 'Mental health conditions include mental disorders and psychosocial disabilities . . . People with mental health conditions are more likely to experience lower levels of mental well-being, but this is not always or necessarily the case.'

This definition seems to imply something about how psychologically robust someone is. Yet it further complicates things, because the term 'mental health' is being used differently here from how it is used elsewhere to mean emotional, psychological and social well-being.[8] 'Mental health' is also commonly used elsewhere as a term to soften language. To say that someone is mentally ill may sound blunt and unkind; by contrast, to say they have poor mental health can remove the stigma of mental suffering. But whilst easier on the ear, the term confuses what is being talked about. This blurring of boundaries and definitions leads to uncertainty in deciding what counts as a problem and who gets to make that judgement.

The emphasis on mental health over recent years has largely been directed towards the milder end of the mental health spectrum. This is not to say that these problems are trivial for the affected individual, but they tend to overlap with what would previously have been considered within the range of normal. I worry about this. Some of the most powerful and effective consultations I have are those in which I am able to tell the individual that their experiences are normal, that to feel that way in response to a life event or situation is a psychologically healthy and normal reaction. Over the years I have come to believe that it often helps to err away from diagnosis rather than towards it. If the wide range of emotions that one can experience are labelled as evidence of poor mental health, it can lead to the unfortunate impression that there must always be something wrong with us if we are experiencing mental anguish. And is there any hope of effective care when there is no longer a consensus on what requires treatment?

Yet mental health is big business. There is a proliferation of wellness and mental health apps. The global market in these apps was estimated to be $6.2 billion in 2023, anticipated to rise by 15.2% per year until 2030.[9] Most people have doubt and hardship in their lives, and are often uncertain how to understand their situation. The apps have started to tap into this insecurity. Our culture has become increasingly one of self-care, which can tip into self-obsession. Put together with a profit motive, this is a recipe for trouble.

The pharmaceutical industry's role in persuading us that we are ill is another factor. Pharmaceutical companies manifestly stand to gain from redefining where the boundaries of normal health lie. If the definitions of depression are loosened, then more antidepressants will be prescribed. One review explored the origins of this loosening of boundaries in the 1960s and 1970s. It highlighted the redefinition of depression in the 1970s from a 'rare and severe psychiatric disorder hitherto treated in asylums' to a 'widespread mild mood disorder to be handled by the general practitioners'.[10] The role of the pharmaceutical industry in promoting this change was evident from the paper. Similarly, where behavioural traits are attributed to ADHD (attention deficit hyperactivity disorder), then it stands to reason that rates of prescription of stimulants will increase. Using pharmaceuticals to treat such problems can often hide the underlying and more complex problems that lie behind a label. And medications are easy to start but much less commonly stopped, even when they don't seem to be providing any benefit. I frequently see people in my clinics who have been treated for years with psychotropic medication on repeat prescription and the initial reason for the prescription lost in the mists of time.

Focus on the milder end of the mental health spectrum may also be taking money away from the less glamorous and too easily forgotten side of mental illness. The increase in referrals that have been generated by expanding rates of diagnosis of mental illness has not been matched by increased resources. As *The Economist* points out,[11] in the past five years there has been a rise of almost one million Britons in contact with mental health services. The figure for seventeen- to nineteen-year-olds with a probable mental health disorder has risen from one in ten to one in four. The same article cites a 22% increase in the overall mental health workforce in the five years to 2021–22 trying to manage a 44% increase in referrals for all patients, leading to an estimated 1.8 million on mental health waiting lists.

Over the same period, the rates of referrals for severe and enduring mental illnesses will have remained the same; diagnoses such as schizophrenia and bipolar disorder are usually hard to miss and not a question of interpretation. Often people with these diagnoses will not actively seek help and are far more costly and resource-intensive to manage well. Yet resources are being spread increasingly thin, and the worry is that money is being diverted away from some of the neediest. The *Economist* article concluded, 'Britain has become more compassionate about mental health. It needs to become more thoughtful, too.' As someone who has spent their professional life delivering care to people suffering from mental illness, I have to agree.

I have hesitated to write this book for fear of being misunderstood. The practice of clinical psychiatry is a complex interplay between science, the reality of people's lives, human nature and pragmatism. I believe in the specialism I have chosen for my career and in the value of high-quality psychiatric care. Over the years, the term 'antipsychiatry' has been used to describe the viewpoint of those who dismiss the whole concept of psychiatric diagnosis. They frame mental illness as a reaction to social problems and the cares of life. To be clear then, I do not support this view. When I meet a new patient who tells me they are suffering in some way, I believe them; but I do not always believe that they have a mental illness. Anyone who has practised clinical psychiatry for any length of time will know that the reality of psychiatric diagnosis is not a question of opinion or debate. Severe depression, anxiety disorders,

OCD, bipolar disorder and schizophrenia, to name only a handful, require skilled and expert management. Yet such serious diseases can get overlooked in the avalanche of new mental health concerns and by medicalising everyday experiences.

This is a challenge to psychiatry as well as to wider society, since at the current rate the number of people who could claim good mental health will be an increasingly small minority, and our capacity to offer treatments to the most severe cases will be compromised as we dilute our precious resources. I believe it is a challenge that needs a response. This book is mine.

2

Psychiatry and Antipsychiatry

The understanding and practice of medicine have changed radically over the centuries. In ancient times, disease was believed to be sent by the gods. Later, Hippocrates (he of the famous Hippocratic oath) believed illnesses were something within the body having gone wrong, rather than the work of spirits or gods.[1] For the most part though, both physical and mental illness were poorly managed. Suffering and poor health were generally accepted by people as their lot, sometimes understood in religious terms as part of a divine plan, with bodily ailments simply something to be endured.[2]

The practice of modern medicine began to take shape in the early twentieth century and accelerated over the course of the century, particularly from the start of the antibiotic era in the 1940s. It heralded a time of increased health expenditure (estimated to be around 1% of GDP in the UK in 1900, 4% in 1970 and 10% in 2015[3]), better evidence on which to base diagnoses, and more effective treatments. Recent decades have seen a further transformation in the understanding of the workings of the body. Diagnosis is supported by imaging and investigations with a precision that a century ago would have been hard to imagine. Yet the human brain and its workings are far more complex and have been much slower to give up their secrets. This has presented

11

challenges to the practice of psychiatry. Whilst the rest of medicine has been able to rely on a greater precision in diagnosis, this has not been available to those studying symptoms of the mind. Psychiatry has therefore remained largely an empirical speciality based on observation and experience. That is not to say it is unscientific – the treatments used are supported by evidence – but it has meant that many of the challenges over the years have been based on a different theoretical understanding of mental suffering, as well as critiques of the way psychiatry has been practised. All of these factors have influenced the current practice of psychiatry.

The period of modern psychiatry can probably be dated to the closing of the asylums in the second half of the twentieth century. Although we now think of asylums as some nightmarish vision of oppression and desperation, their original intention was a noble one. They were places where mentally ill people who were destitute, downtrodden and, all too frequently, abused were offered a place of refuge. They were asylums in the true meaning of the word.

Prior to asylums, the vast majority of people with mental illness were cared for at home, or not cared for at all and living on the streets. In the mid-eighteenth century there were only three public asylums, although after the 1808 County Asylums Act, and for the next 150 years, the number of asylums steadily grew.[4] They were initially built outside towns, where fresh air and a more congenial environment were part of the therapeutic intervention. Yet for most of the asylum era, effective treatments for mental illness were still decades away, which made it difficult to discharge inmates. Inevitably the population swelled, and by 1954 around 150,000 people were living in an asylum in the UK.[4]

The end of the asylum era was the result of a confluence of factors. One of them was the development of effective drugs to treat mental illness. The first antipsychotic was developed in a French pharmaceutical laboratory in 1951. Initially designed as a drug that might help in general anaesthesia,[5] it was discovered by chance to have an effect on symptoms of psychosis such as delusional beliefs and hallucinations. By 1952, chlorpromazine had become the first available antipsychotic on the market, and by 1955 its use was widespread throughout the world.[5]

Having this effective treatment for the symptoms of illnesses such as schizophrenia was transformative. It meant that many of those in asylums who had a psychotic illness became well enough to be discharged and start to live independently. Chlorpromazine is still going strong, by the way. Over seventy years later, it is still licensed and used in the treatment of schizophrenia and other psychotic illnesses.

Chlorpromazine wasn't the only major breakthrough from that decade. Antidepressants were also developed in the 1950s, the first being iproniazid. This, like chlorpromazine, was a fortuitous discovery.[6] It was intended as a medication to treat tuberculosis, but its side effects of euphoria and improved sleep led to its trial as an antidepressant. At the same time, another type of antidepressant, imipramine, was developed (another drug still used today). These discoveries began a new era of effective treatments for patients. In fact, they heralded a golden age of discovery for psychiatric drugs over the following decades.

Alongside the discovery of new medications, there was a political movement away from institutionalised care and towards care in the community, not least because of the potential cost saving. In 1961, the health minister Enoch Powell announced his intention to close down the asylums. His aim was to cut the provision of asylum beds by at least 75,000 (about half of all beds), to go 'as low as we dare, perhaps lower'. In knocking down the asylum buildings, he said, 'it is our duty to err on the side of ruthlessness'.[7]

The third reason for the closure of the asylums was the most challenging for psychiatry. It came about through the counter-culture social movement of the 1960s and 1970s. Criticism of the asylums had been building from both inside and outside psychiatry. One of the best known came in the form of a book called *Asylums*, written by American sociologist Erving Goffman.[8] Going undercover in an asylum, playing the role of assistant to the athletics director, he made careful observations of daily life, and the result was devastating. Referring to asylums as 'total institutions', he observed 'a place of residence and work where a large number of like-situated individuals, cut off from the wider society for an appreciable period of time, together lead an enclosed, formally administered round of life'.[8] He described the way in which staff and inmates lived in different worlds, the staff working eight-hour shifts, whilst the inmates were stuck there for twenty-four hours a day. Worse were the antagonism and mutual suspicion. Staff felt themselves to be 'superior and righteous', whilst the inmates considered themselves 'inferior, weak, blameworthy and guilty'. Strangely, the thing that spoke to me most in Goffman's descriptions was the feeling of drift and boredom. The patients living in the asylum had little to differentiate their days, no leisure time, family time or work time as in most people's lives. For the inmates of the asylums, there was just time. There were no decisions to be made, no goals to strive for, just the stultifying conformity of their formally administered lives. Goffman described the gradual way in which the will to rebel against the system was extinguished. Eventually, inmates accepted their situation, in a process that became known as institutionalisation. The goal of treatment should be self-reliance and independence, but the asylums had brought about the opposite. There was little about these places that was therapeutic. Goffman's critique was powerful, and its influence on psychiatry, particularly the closure of institutions, was significant.

Goffman was thrust into what quickly became known as the antipsychiatry movement. This is not a term that he or the others included under the label accepted, but it stuck. The criticism of this movement was levelled not just at the practice of psychiatry, such as the asylums, but at the very validity of psychiatry as a discipline. One of the most prominent critics was Thomas Szasz, a psychoanalyst whose most famous work, *The Myth of Mental Illness*, was published in 1961. In a paper of the same name, he began his introduction with the provocative statement: 'My aim in this essay is to raise the question "Is there such a thing as mental illness?" and to argue that there is not.'[9]

Szasz considered that problems diagnosed as mental illness were actually related to the problems and pressures of life. He saw the label of mental illness as a distraction from the real issues, which were, he said, the problems of living. He argued that psychiatric diagnoses were simply labels used to describe anyone who had symptoms that deviated from societal norms. Given his belief that there was no such thing as mental illness, it followed that he would view psychiatric intervention as coercive and wrong-headed.

Whilst modern psychiatry posited that the root cause of mental illness was some part of the brain having gone awry, Szasz disagreed. He did not see mental illness as a 'real' illness like neurological illness, in which a scan would show which bit of the nervous system has been affected. Interesting though his argument was, it could not account for the fact that some illnesses accepted as neurological, such as migraine, have no neatly explainable cause that can be observed in the brain. And the converse is also true: some clear-cut brain diseases, such as neurosyphilis, give rise to mental problems. But then he argued that if a psychiatric symptom could be traced back to the brain, it was no longer a mental disease but a neurological disease, a kind of checkmate for psychiatry.

Another vocal critic of psychiatry was Scottish psychiatrist, R. D. Laing, who argued for something similar to Szasz. He saw mental illness as a social construct, rather than something real. His best-known work, *The Divided Self*, was published in 1960. He believed that schizophrenia was, in the words of one commentary 'an understandable, even normal, response . . . of sensitive individuals to a mad world'.[10] In this way, he argued, symptoms of schizophrenia were not meaningless rantings but carried some essential information that would help the patient make sense of what was going on. Guided by an interested healer, who was able to listen carefully to the content of what they were saying, they would be led through the thicket of their life situation and back to normality.

One social theory of mental illness even managed to blame the patient's mother for the problem of their offspring. This was the infamous 'schizophrenogenic mother'.[11] The theory went that schizophrenia may have been the result of some unfortunate personality type that the mother had. And so, in some clinics, mothers were given personality tests to winkle out what may have led to their unfortunate child developing schizophrenia.[11] It was also suggested that schizophrenia could be caused by mixed messages given to the child; for example, the mother being both over-protective and rejecting the child.[12] If having a child with schizophrenia did not present enough problems in the mother's life, blaming them for it too would surely have pushed some over the edge.

Problems for psychiatry continued to mount. In 1973, psychologist David Rosenhan conducted an experiment that had the psychiatric world rocking on its heels.[13] The design of the pseudopatient experiment was simple. Eight individuals were instructed to get themselves admitted to a psychiatric institution by telling the doctors they were having auditory hallucinations.

They were instructed to say that they heard the words 'empty,' 'hollow' and 'thud'. Once admitted, the pseudopatients were instructed to behave normally and be fully cooperative with staff and ward procedures. When asked how they were once they were on the ward, they were told to say that they were feeling fine. The pseudopatients were also told they needed to convince the staff that they were sane in order to be discharged – as for any other patient admitted to a psychiatric ward.

Once the pseudopatients were on the ward, Rosenhan discovered that even normal behaviour, such as writing, was seen through a lens of pathology. As one example, they had been instructed by the experimenter to take extensive notes whilst on the ward. Yet in some cases, without being asked what they were writing about, the nurse would record that the 'patient engages in writing behaviour'.[13] All the patients were eventually discharged (some after seven days, some not for fifty-two days, with an average of nineteen days) and all were given a diagnosis of 'schizophrenia in remission'.

In a kind of inverse to the one described above, a second experiment was performed. This time, the hospitals were warned to expect pseudopatients to secretly turn up to their departments. Of 193 patients attending various departments, forty-one were thought, with a high degree of confidence by at least one member of staff, to be a pseudopatient. In nineteen cases this judgement was made by a psychiatrist too.[13] As it turned out, no pseudopatients had been instructed to turn up, and (at least as far as the authors knew) all of the patients were real and genuinely seeking help.

With these two experiments, the psychiatric profession had been charged and found guilty of being unable to differentiate normality from mental illness. The impact on the profession was significant. Psychiatry has always had a capacity for self-reflection, and much of the criticism that followed was from psychiatrists themselves. There was a realisation that things had to change. Yet even at the time, some were voicing serious questions about the validity of the original Rosenhan experiment, including Robert Spitzer, one of the most highly regarded psychiatrists of his generation. Spitzer would later go on to chair the task force that developed DSM-III, the third incarnation of the diagnostic bible, the version that was the start of the modern classification systems of psychiatric disease.

Spitzer described the Rosenhan paper as 'pseudoscience presented as science'[14] and took it apart from its foundations. He argued that admitting someone claiming to have auditory hallucinations might not be a sign of something wrong with the psychiatric profession, but rather believing the patient's distress. He added that although the patients were given instructions to talk only about auditory hallucinations, even in 1973 (when the experiment took place) you would need a bit more than that to get admitted. He surmises that the pseudopatients would have had to pretend to be distressed by their mental experiences to get admitted. He went on to say that they did not, as claimed, behave normally once on the ward. 'Normal' would have been to tell one of the nurses that they had got themselves admitted as part of an experiment, show the proof of this and leave the ward. And finally, he pointed out that to be discharged with a diagnosis of 'schizophrenia in remission' was so vanishingly rare that it almost never happened. The psychiatrists would have been able to see that whatever problems the pseudopatients may initially have experienced had, unusually, resolved entirely during the course of the admission.

There is a footnote to this whole episode. In 2023, half a century after the original Rosenhan paper, another paper was published. It had a title that left little room for doubt: 'Rosenhan revisited: successful scientific fraud'.[15] The paper, written by medical historian Andrew Scull, is based on the findings of journalist Susannah Cahalan. Calling Rosenhan's paper 'a spectacularly successful case of scientific fraud', Scull takes apart the Rosenhan study. As had been suspected, the pseudopatients had done a lot more to convince the admitting psychiatrist they were mentally ill than reporting hallucinations using the words 'empty,' 'hollow' and 'thud'. In fact, it turned out that Rosenhan himself was one of the pseudopatients, and when his admission notes were tracked down, they painted a very different picture. He told the admitting psychiatrist he was able to hear other people's thoughts, so that he had to put copper over his ears to shut them out. He admitted to suicidal thoughts and an inability to work because of his symptoms. The psychiatrist added in his notes that the patient appeared to be perplexed and frightened.[15]

Attention was drawn to many other flaws and inconsistencies in Rosenhan's paper. Most of the patients could not be tracked down, and the ones that were found gave a different version of their experience. A significant feature of Rosenhan's study was how little meaningful patient contact there had been, but the patients either didn't record how long staff had spent with them or recalled that there had been a lot of individualised contact. There was apparent tampering with statistics, a lack of verifiable raw data and little evidence that the diagnosis of 'schizophrenia in remission' was actually unwarranted in the cases where this was made[15] based on the information available to the treating psychiatrist.

In spite of everything we now know, the Rosenhan paper is still widely cited, and its effects are still evident today. It is hard to think of a single paper that has been more influential on the self-image and practice of psychiatry. And yet, it is notable that this attack, like others of its era, came on the crest of the counterculture movement, and the criticisms of both psychiatric diagnosis and its clinical practice reflected that time. They came from a humanistic perspective. The objections to psychiatry and its diagnostic lexicon were rooted in the philosophical. Was there such a thing as mental illness? And if there were symptoms that might be ascribed to mental illness, wasn't that just the rational response of sensitive people living in a crazy world?

There was also an emphasis on freedom, autonomy and liberalism. Szasz and others saw the practice of psychiatry as coercive and illiberal. Psychiatry, they believed, forced people to accept treatment for diagnoses that weren't real, to manage symptoms or behaviours that society found inconvenient or deviant. In this respect, psychiatry was seen as little more than an agent of social control, acting on behalf of the state rather than the patients it purported to treat. The opposition to psychiatry was expressed plainly and even forcefully, yet one sensed from the literature that there was little personal hostility. Fundamentally, all sides were doing what they felt was in the best interest of the unfortunate individuals suffering mental anguish.

Over the years, opposition to psychiatry has evolved. It has become angrier, more personalised. It is more diffuse and the criticisms less coherent. They are no longer based on a philosophical objection to psychiatric diagnosis. Or at least, not only that. Today, there are a range of issues, with the emphasis depending on the particular objective of the people or organisations attacking psychiatry.

A recent phenomenon has been alternative, evidence-based readings of the science. If research evidence could be shown to prove that established treatments in psychiatry don't work, it is argued, it would follow that the authority of psychiatry would be seriously undermined.

This can be seen in the energetic opposition to electroconvulsive therapy (ECT). It is a treatment that has never been popular.

Despite the reality of modern ECT taking place under general anaesthetic and lasting for around a minute or two, it sounds barbaric. It has become a touchstone issue. It is true that there are alternative, pharmaceutical treatments now that can help in many, but not all, cases. And as a treatment of last resort, used only in the more desperate or life-threatening cases of depression, it has been proved to be effective. The vast body of evidence would support the use of ECT for select cases. It is approved by the National Institute for Health and Care Excellence in the UK and the Food and Drug Administration in the US.[16] It is not without side effects. In particular, it can affect memory, and this is not a trivial problem, so the pros and cons must be carefully weighed in each case. But when ECT is used, it is always because the alternatives of not offering this treatment to the patient are even worse.

Some of the discussion about the efficacy of ECT may have been informed by the way it was used in the past, or perhaps by ideas about a future in which there will be other effective treatments available, and this is understandable. But for some who criticise it, there is an ideological dimension. It seems that to concede that ECT works is to admit that there is something 'real' about depression. If you take the view that depression is a socially constructed illness, then ECT shouldn't alleviate the symptoms – and if that is your starting point, then selective readings of the published literature will always lead to the conclusion you want. But that's not how science is meant to be. When your starting point for the assessment of data is your own conclusions, it is bad for science and can only be harmful to patients.

It is easy to criticise from the sidelines, or to consider the situation in abstract terms, but a psychiatrist managing the care of a patient catatonic with depression, neither eating or drinking or even talking, in the very depths of unimaginable mental pain, must judge how best to use the tools at hand. Nobody loves having to perform ECT, any more than a surgeon would love having to amputate a diseased limb, but we live in the real world, where difficult decisions about treatment have to be made. I can think of several cases I have been involved in where ECT has proved to be life-saving.

ECT is not the only treatment for depression that has been the subject of debates, which are as frequently played out on social media as in the scientific literature. The current battleground is about the effectiveness of a class of antidepressant medications called selective serotonin reuptake inhibitors (SSRIs), which increase the neurochemical serotonin in the brain. They are the most pre-scribed antidepressants in the UK. One argument against the medications has been that we do not, when it really comes down to it, know exactly how they work, or why increasing serotonin in the brain helps to treat depression. Yet the same argument could be made of other medications, including paracetamol,[17] one of the most widely prescribed drugs in the world, and general anaesthet-ics,[18] which also have somewhat mysterious mechanisms of action. Yet no opposition exists to these drugs. Psychiatry just seems to be held to different standards.

When I was a psychiatry trainee, I worked for a professor of psychopharmacology, who died tragically young. He was shy, kind, far from a natural at small talk, but razor sharp. One day we were in his office, discussing the mechanism of action of psychotropic medications, in other words, entirely in his comfort zone. The actual way these drugs worked to cure psychosis, when I pressed him on it, turned out to be a little hazy. 'Al,' he said to me, 'Just because beta blockers are used in the treatment of angina, it doesn't mean that angina is caused by something wrong with your beta receptors.'

The point was well taken. We know that angina is caused by a partial blockage in your coronary arteries. Beta blockers help to control the symptoms, but they are nothing to do with what caused it. Similarly, when we take paracetamol to treat a headache, nobody is saying the headache is caused by paracetamol deficiency. Whatever serotonin is doing in treating depression, we don't fully know. But we do have plenty of evidence from clinical trials that these types of medication work.

Yet there is still a disproportionate opposition to medications like antidepressants, and alternative readings of the science. Just like for ECT, there are facts, alternative facts and alternative interpretations of those facts. What are the public meant to think? How do they know which version to believe? I have had patients stop their antidepressant medication because of media reporting of the issue, to the overall detriment of their care. I understand the patients' position, and I don't blame the media either, who are generally trying to report complexity as best they can. But I can't think of any other medical speciality where there is the same level of opposition to treatments likely to help patients, based on ideological reasons as much as any analysis of the research literature. Some of the criticism of antidepressants comes from within psychiatry. I have no issue with this. As for any profession, criticism can improve the practice of it. But psychiatrists have collectively reviewed the data, assessed the evidence and concluded that antidepressants are undoubtedly effective.

Some of the criticism against psychiatry comes from professions that are allied to it, in what can start to feel like a kind of guild warfare. This goes beyond just antidepressants. In a move reminiscent of Laing and Szasz from a bygone era, some have rejected the concept of diagnosis. An alternative system to understand patients' distress has been proposed, known as the Power Threat Meaning Framework. The underlying idea is that mental illness is a reflection of power imbalance, such as poverty or an abusive relationship. This imbalance carries a threat to individuals on the wrong end of it, who will react to this threat in ways that might appear to be mental illness but aren't. According to this theory, what appears to be mental illness may be the appropriate reactions to societal injustice, power imbalances and other social adversity.[19]

Yet if this framework is intended to replace diagnosis, where is the evidence that the totality of what we understand as mental illness – including schizophrenia and bipolar disorder – is nothing more than a reaction to adversity? We will see over the course of this book psychiatry's difficulties with defining the boundaries of diagnosis. But to throw out the whole concept of diagnosis in favour of a theory for which there is no evidence does not seem to represent progress.

The Power Threat Meaning Framework also misses another issue, which is that psychiatrists have long understood mental illness to be a combination of the biological (genetics, brain chemistry and neuronal wiring), psychological (thinking patterns, often learned through experience) and social (poverty, racism, abuse amongst others). Open any textbook of psychiatry written in the last fifty years and you will see, written somewhere in the introduction, that psychiatry is a bio-psycho-social speciality. In truth, so is any other medical speciality. Heart attacks might be because someone is predisposed to high cholesterol and diabetes. But not that alone; they also smoke, live unhealthily, have stressful jobs and lives. Social factors play a role in the whole of medicine, including in mental illness, but psychiatry seems to be singled out for opposition to its method of diagnosis and treatment. In 2016, there was even a Scholarship in Antipsychiatry created at the University of Toronto for students working on this topic.[20] I don't think any of us will live to see the day that an anticardiology scholarship is created at any university.

There is one other important constituency who are against psychiatry, and these are the patients who have either been harmed by psychiatry or believe that they have been harmed by it. And here I would have to say that psychiatrists have not always been quick to acknowledge the potential harms our treatments have caused. Patients told us about memory problems caused by ECT for some time before this was fully investigated and accepted. Similarly, some patients talked about the difficulties they have had in coming off antidepressants, with unpleasant discontinuation symptoms, before this was more formally addressed by the profession. Currently, there is a discussion about whether a small minority of patients have persistent sexual side effects after taking a certain class of antidepressants, and it is important for psychiatrists to listen rather than to dismiss them as minor, trivial or rare. I believe psychiatry has done a great deal of good for a great many people, but how could psychiatrists not acknowledge the people who have been let down? And who might not feel animosity if they had been let down in this way, their concerns unacknowledged and inadequate support given?

I would also recognise that care of patients on inpatient wards has not always been therapeutic. They have often been crowded, stressful places to be. And the side effects of antipsychotic medications have, for many patients, been a heavy price to pay for the treatment of their psychotic illness. In this respect, what might be considered part of the antipsychiatry movement is, in fact, a consumerist movement. People have tried what psychiatry has had to offer and found it wanting. Patients with psychotic illnesses like schizophrenia are amongst the most marginalised, vulnerable and damaged individuals in our society, and I have wondered if we could, should have done better.

Many of the criticisms of psychiatry have been understandable and important, and some have been made with different agendas. It is important, though, to listen to them. Psychiatry as a profession has always had a capacity for self-reflection and has grown from the debates over the years. Questions are at the heart of psychiatric practice. This is the case within the clinical consultation, where each day I ask a great number of questions to my patients, trying to better understand their mental experiences. And in the wider historical context of the practice of psychiatry, questions about what diagnoses are, what their value is, how we conceptualise them and how robust they are, are all crucial too.

3

A Diagnostic Dilemma

Many years ago, I was on holiday in the US. It was in the 1980s, at a time when the intrusion of advertising into every corner of life was, for me at least, an amusing novelty (although in retrospect, it was also a warning from the future). One afternoon, driving along the never-ending miles of freeway, another advertisement came on the radio. The scene was set. A woman is sitting on a crowded bus, somewhere in a downtown suburban city. She opens her handbag. A whoof of fetid handbag air escapes to her great consternation, and to the disgust of the other passengers. The moment freezes. 'Do you have purse odour?' asks the voiceover, which was at once accusing and sympathetic. We realise that opening her purse in public has caused the woman terrific embarrassment. I imagine her losing friends as they dissociate themselves from someone who is prepared to use a malodorous purse. And just like that, a diagnosis had come into being: purse odour. For which, happily, the solution was something companies both had and were prepared to sell to you. I don't exactly remember what the cure was now, but I recall it as a scented little bag to slip inside your purse, reminding me of the way medieval doctors carried aromatic herbs inside their plague masks, to prevent infection from entering their bodies. In this way, purse odour had developed a reality. The manufacturers were able to describe a problem, formulate a diagnosis and then offer a cure.

I have thought since about that advertisement. Of course, handbags don't have diagnoses in the way that people do, but as an analogy for diagnoses, it made me wonder how it would stand up. On the one hand, everybody understands that a problem has been created for the purpose of selling the solution. Yet it has arrived in a time and place where the main concerns for many are no longer hunger or homelessness, but rather the minutiae of navigating modern life. Handbag odour would never have troubled a cutpurse in medieval England, hiding in the bushes to commit an act of highway robbery. It is an invented diagnosis that, if it could be described as a problem at all, is a very contemporary one.

On the other hand, in an environment where social embarrassment ranks highly, the thought of other people being disgusted by you, or them thinking of your handbag or purse as disagreeable, or seeing it as an off-putting reflection of you, is not necessarily trivial. It might not have been relevant 800 years ago, but that isn't the point. Social embarrassment and shame are real, and a powerful motivator.

How diagnoses are conceptualised and understood is of the utmost importance in modern psychiatry. It is the framework on which psychiatry is built. I would contend that psychiatry is a far better discipline because of them. Diagnoses are also imperfect. This in itself does not detract from their legitimacy. Perfection is not possible to achieve in psychiatric diagnosis. For a start, there is (at least currently) no external validator like changes on a brain scan or blood test results. If we compare neurology and psychiatry, the difference is that neurological illnesses are diseases of the brain and so are usually measurable on scans or by other diagnostic tools. Psychiatric illnesses are diseases of the mind, and so cannot. Yet even this distinction does not hold up to scrutiny. Many neurological illnesses, such as Parkinson's disease, have psychiatric symptoms (hence the speciality of neuropsychiatry in which I work). And by contrast, some illnesses thought to be primarily psychiatric have turned out to have clear-cut organic causes. This has led to some calls for the distinction between psychiatry and neurology to be abandoned. In fact, one commentary from senior neuropsychiatrists concluded that 'there is no implicit hierarchy in what emerges as the brain-based hallmark of neurological versus psychiatric conditions; they both involve the functionally interesting parts of the brain, it is just that they are, quite subtly, different'.[1]

Kenneth Kendler, one of the doyens of modern psychiatry, provides an excellent overview of the philosophical underpinnings of psychiatric diagnosis,[2] and several of his ideas are incorporated into the frameworks here. The starting point for understanding psychiatric diagnosis can be simplified (or more accurately oversimplified) into two opposing views. The first view would say that psychiatric diagnoses are real entities. They exist in nature, independently of doctors or psychiatrists. In this way, you could consider them much like gravity. They are out there, waiting to be discovered, and if they are not discovered, they will still exist. In this view, diagnoses in our classification systems, such as the International Classification of Diseases (ICD) and DSM, are simply describing an existing reality.

The opposing view is that psychiatric diagnoses are not real but invented, constructed like purse odour. The argument would go that there is nothing natural about diagnoses, they are not real entities and they do not exist 'out there' in the world just waiting to be discovered. This 'constructivist' view would be that diagnoses are simply made up. Looking at it this way, they can be seen as a means for societies to delineate the boundaries of normal behaviour and control or marginalise people who fall outside those boundaries.

Whilst both the 'realist' and 'constructivist' arguments contain something of truth in them, neither is quite adequate to the task of understanding diagnosis in psychiatry. If we think back to purse odour and we were to advance it as a diagnosis, we would say that it exists as a socially constructed diagnosis. It does not have any real existence outside of that society, and we could easily imagine a world in which that diagnosis did not exist. This is unlike schizophrenia, for example, which would exist in any society, whatever we decided to call it. We understand, however, that different patients can present with different symptoms of schizophrenia. It is not quite as reproducible as gravity. Yet between these two opposites, 'real' and 'constructed', there are other ways of understanding how a diagnostic category in psychiatry is arrived at.

A paper written by Dutch psychologist Denny Borsboom articulates what many of us intuitively understand to be true: that behaviours and symptoms exist on a continuum in a population. He refers to this as a dimensional perspective.[3] Although not without its own drawbacks, at its most straightforward the theory would be that individuals have an inherent susceptibility to develop a particular symptom or group of symptoms. Take depression as an example. There are a number of symptoms of depression, which are experienced by most of us at one time or other in our lives. Having a couple of them at a given time doesn't make you depressed. You need to have enough of them to reach the threshold for a diagnosis. As individuals, we also have a greater or lesser susceptibility to those symptoms developing. Some people develop depression with minimal triggers or none at all. Most of us would develop symptoms of depression if faced with enough adversity. When someone develops a certain number of these typical depressive symptoms, then we may categorise them as depressed. We may go on to say that they have mild, moderate or severe depression, depending on the number and intensity of symptoms. The choice of how many symptoms are needed for the threshold for depression to be reached, or what makes a mild case as opposed to a moderate or severe case, is decided through careful observation and research, and by committees of experts. In this continuum model, the diagnosis is real – and nobody would seriously dispute that depression is not real – but the thresholds to make the diagnosis are not precisely scientific, even if thoughtfully considered.

Kendler adds another category of socially influenced diagnosis.[2] These are diagnoses in which symptoms may have been commonly experienced, but for whatever reason were not acknowledged as diagnoses until the social climate allowed for them to be so. He gives as an example the inclusion of premenstrual dysphoric disorder (PMDD) in DSM-5. This disorder will be familiar to many women, although it began its life as premenstrual syndrome (PMS). It was later called the slightly less snappily titled 'luteal phase dysphoric disorder' (LPDD), so called because the symptoms are primarily experienced in the luteal phase of the menstrual cycle, that phase beginning after ovulation and before menstruation, and start to improve in the days after menses begins. Typical symptoms of PMDD include bloating, breast tenderness, mood swings, anxiety and irritability, as well as changes in sleep and appetite.

PMDD is undoubtedly describing something real. It is its classification as a psychiatric diagnosis that has been controversial. One paper published a summary of the discussions and arguments that took place prior to its inclusion in the DSM diagnostic classification.[4] A powerful argument against its inclusion was that women's bodies, particularly in relation to their reproductive systems, have over centuries been subjected to a male-dominated and patriarchal medical perspective. Hysteria was considered to be a female affliction caused by a wandering womb. Puberty, menstruation and menopause were believed to put repeated strains on the female body, thereby weakening it. As Andrew Scull writes in his biography of hysteria,[5] women were seen as inferior versions of men ('moister, looser textured, softer with spongier flesh') and so their bodies liable to break down under the continued pressures of their reproductive system.

In this context, the inclusion as a psychiatric disorder of symptoms related to what is a normal female experience, menstruation, was an affront to many, who saw PMDD as the pathologising of something normal and natural.[4,6] And given that the symptoms include many physical ones (bloating, breast tenderness, sleep difficulties) rather than just psychiatric ones (irritability, anxiety, mood swings), its inclusion within the category of mental disorders was an added provocation. It suggested that women experiencing symptoms, even in the luteal phase of their menstrual cycles, could be seen (and diagnosed) as mentally unwell, just as they had in earlier phases of medical history.

The opposing view was that accurate identification of symptoms such as PMDD would legitimise a fairly common experience, estimated to affect around 1.2–6.4% of women.[7] In this context, the inclusion of PMDD would be seen as a sign that women were finally being listened to and taken seriously. Premenstrual symptoms are real and distressing, rather than an excuse, the punchline of a joke or something to be brushed aside. As Kendler points out,[2] PMDD's inclusion in DMS was partly down to a social change. Women were more readily able to accept their menstrual symptoms without embarrassment, and expect that they would be taken seriously. This acceptance, driven by women themselves, helped to ease the transition of PMDD into the formal psychiatric lexicon.

But there were also other factors in play. One of these was pharmaceutical-led. Evidence emerged that PMDD symptoms were improved by SSRIs. These included the best known of all these antidepressants, fluoxetine, which had spent most of its life marketed as Prozac. Now, with treatment of PMDD opening a new seam for its prescription, it was renamed Sarafem and packaged as a lavender and pink tablet.[6] Once the US Federal Drug Administration approved Sarafem for use in PMDD, it became all but impossible to resist the inclusion of PMDD in the diagnostic manuals, since it was now a diagnosable and treatable disorder. That the diagnosis was a bit loose, and of uncertain diagnostic validity, did not stop its inclusion, because the available evidence supported the treatment.

One final argument was also advanced for its inclusion. If it was a diagnosis, it could be studied as such, and attract research funding.[4] This, the argument went, would lead to improved ways of understanding PMDD and managing it too, to the overall benefit of women affected by the symptoms.

PMDD existed before psychiatric classifications existed, and its symptoms will still be there even if it is removed from the classification systems. In that respect, it is not a social construct, but as Kendler comments, its inclusion and conceptualisation as a diagnosis are new and undoubtedly socially influenced.[2] I can see both sides of the argument for its inclusion in DSM-5. Instinctively, my sympathies are for the argument against its inclusion. I have worried for too long about diagnostic creep, whereby the category of normal is consistently eroded. I also have concerns about a situation in which symptoms associated with menstruation are pathologised. But as a practising clinician, if a woman comes to see me with severe PMDD symptoms that are causing problems in her life, it is hard to ignore the reality of it. And crucially, it is even harder to justify treating it with medication if it is not recognised as a diagnosis, because psychiatric drugs are typically licensed to treat diagnoses, not symptoms.

Another way of thinking about the construct of psychiatric

diagnosis is what Borsboom refers to as causal systems and Kendler as homeostatic property clusters.[2, 3] This is a kind of third way between saying that diagnoses are entities that exist in nature that we have discovered (like gravity) and that they are socially constructed (like purse odour). This third way postulates that there are networks of symptoms that are interrelated. For example, paranoia may make someone think that they are being followed. This might lead to elaborate behaviours such as covering windows and keyholes in the house to avoid the chance of being spied on at home. The persistent fear of being monitored leads to social withdrawal, which in turn may start to cause depressive symptoms, and the cumulative effects of it all leading to suicidal thoughts. In this way, a whole networked system of symptoms and behaviours becomes evident.

In this respect, as Borsboom argues, when we are measuring the number of symptoms someone has to decide whether they qualify for a diagnosis, we may be measuring something real about how many of these networked systems have been activated, and hence provide some measure of severity of the illness in question. This concept may also explain the overlap between different diagnoses, because some of the same networks, for example, insomnia and paranoia, may be triggered in different conditions. In short, there are various ways of understanding psychiatric diagnoses, all philosophically and conceptually a little different, and, importantly, all of which can be true simultaneously for different conditions and at different times.

There is also a further dimension to psychiatric diagnosis, which has little to do with the philosophical considerations above. It is about how diagnoses get used in the real world. How might a particular diagnosis, handed down from a set of guidelines, get used? I have often thought that before new diagnostic classification systems are released for general use in psychiatry, consideration should be given to how they might go wrong – what you could think of as an ante-mortem, rather than the usual post-mortem that happens after it's all too late. Because the fact is that the language of mental illness is increasingly used in ways that bear no relation to the meaning that the diagnosis originally had.

This has been called a 'looping effect'.[8] It describes the ways in which diagnoses frame how people think about their suffering. In turn, people interact with diagnoses to alter the criteria on which they are made, in a kind of feedback loop. One paper,[9] for example, explored how adolescents took ownership of their diagnosis of depression or anxiety, defining it in different terms from their doctors and using it to describe different things. For example, the paper describes how young people might use the terms 'anxiety' and 'depression' to describe feeling low, with anxiety 'given various meanings such as having too much to do, being uncertain or aware that one might not succeed, or having to do things they did not really feel like doing'. The authors summarised the paper by saying that the 'participants [of the study] gave new meaning to these psychiatric labels, devalued and gave nuance to them, and by doing so transformed them into cultural categories rather than diagnostic categories'.[9]

The consequences of such looping effects are that diagnoses become looser – the way in which a diagnosis is commonly used in the public square feeds back into how that particular diagnosis is made in the future. In the case of depression, it may be that only two or three symptoms suffice to make a diagnosis, whereas previously it might have been five or six. Or it may also be that other, milder criteria would now allow someone to qualify for a diagnosis. Similarly, the criteria needed now for a diagnosis of autism have led to a substantial increase in the number of people diagnosed. And as the number of people diagnosed with a particular condition rises, the feedback loop can start to change the criteria used to make the diagnosis.

This has happened by degrees across a range of different diagnoses, and each time with good intentions. We have been more inclusive with respect to diagnosis, chipped away at the borders, made sure that everyone is properly diagnosed and treated. We have reduced stigma, at least for certain diagnoses, so that people are generally more willing to accept a diagnostic label. And I think for some people, who are struggling for an identity or a way to make sense of their lives, a diagnostic label can help provide one.

Mental health awareness campaigns have, despite the best of intentions, added to the impression that psychiatric diagnoses are everywhere. There is evidence that talking about mental health disorders increases the rates of people identifying with them. In their paper, Foulkes and Andrews argue that awareness raising leads to people interpreting milder symptoms as mental health problems, which can lead to behaviour changes and compound the symptoms they experience. This, multiplied throughout a population, increases the rates of the disorder being diagnosed, which in turn can lead to more awareness campaigns.[10] And so the cycle continues. It is not hard to conclude that, in trying to be kind and inclusive, we have inadvertently done harm to individuals and populations. In fact, I would contend that most people with mental illness already know that there is something wrong. Their reluctance to come forward for treatment is not for lack of awareness, but about whether the right help is out there. The solution is not to raise awareness but to provide adequate services. Yet the paradox of awareness raising is that it increases the number who need, or feel that they need, mental health support, thus making it decreasingly available.

Psychiatry has to navigate these models of understanding of illness and disease in a shifting cultural landscape. There is an inherent imprecision in this, so there is a need for judgement, not only in diagnosis but also in how it is communicated. Whether treatments are offered and what type of treatments they will be (whether that be psychotropic medication, talking therapies or social care) must also be navigated in the context of the particular social environment that exists at that time.

Of course, psychiatry is not the only medical speciality that has to factor in the changing cultural climate when making diagnoses or recommending treatments. For many medical diagnoses, there is still a lack of precision. Discussions about these diagnoses, often the subject of debate in the media and on social media, echo those that take place with psychiatric diagnoses. Fibromyalgia and ME, to name just a couple of examples, lack a clear understanding of the underlying pathology. They are defined by their symptoms, rather than by any blood test or scan. And inevitably this has led to some of the same questions about whether they are 'real' diagnoses or constructed.

Yet perhaps the biggest change that all doctors have had to navigate, whether within psychiatry or the rest of medicine, is a change in the doctor–patient dynamic. There has been a fundamental shift in our social attitudes towards medical authority and the ownership of knowledge, and this also impacts how diagnoses are made or, perhaps now more accurately, how diagnoses are agreed with patients. When I think back, this is a process that has been changing over years. The first exam I ever failed was in my first year at medical school. It was a sociology exam. I remember the question clearly. 'In the doctor–patient relationship, both the doctor and the patient are experts. Discuss.'

I made a trenchant, uncompromising case for the doctor being the actual expert, whilst the patient's role was merely the grateful recipient of the doctor's wisdom. Had I been taking the exam in 1950, no doubt I would have scored very highly. Looking back,

I think my answer simply reflected my own unquestioning faith in the authority of doctors. But even by the mid-1980s, when I took that exam, there was a recognition that the roles of the doctor and patient had changed; they were now a complementary relationship. This involved an elevation of the patient's role, as having an expertise in their own symptoms and illness and, particularly for long-term illnesses, their own diagnosis. This allowed for a more equal relationship between doctors and patients as partners in medical care.

Had I been taking that exam now, my answer would have been very different. The democratisation of information is, of course, a good thing. A well-informed public can only enhance care. Yet this is only really going to work if there is a shared understanding of the human body and how it functions. We are still some way off this goal. In times gone by, patients were often deliberately kept in the dark about aspects of their illness and its treatment. Oliver Wendell Holmes, in a lecture given to a graduating medical school class in 1871, said, 'Your patient has no more right to all the truth than he has to all the medicine in your saddle-bags . . . he should get only just so much as is good for him.'[11]

In the early post-antibiotic days of the 1950s, there still remained a significant differential of knowledge between patients and their medical practitioners. This was in the days before search engines, computers or readily accessible knowledge. In my very first week as a medical student in 1986, I was shown a study published in 1970[12] that asked patients what they understood by commonly used medical terms and how they understood their bodies. The results of patients were compared with those of doctors who had been asked to complete the same questions. The lecturer wanted to illustrate that as the workings of the human body became second nature to us as we progressed through medical school, it was easy to forget what the average person knew, or even what we knew now. As one learns things, they have a way of becoming obvious to us. 'Palpitations' were understood by all of the doctors in the study to be a feeling of the heart thumping inside the chest, whereas amongst members of the public (patients who happened to be attending an outpatient clinic), many thought they were feelings of breathlessness, a feeling of fright or panic, or a pain in the chest over the heart.

What sticks in my memory most about that study, however, was the slide that the lecturer showed. There were four panels. In each panel was a diagram of the outline of a man with the kidneys placed in a different location in the body. Only one of the four diagrams had the correct kidney location. Patients were asked to say in which panel the kidneys were in the correct anatomical position. It turned out that less than half of the people asked knew where their kidneys were, with the rest locating the kidneys in the chest, groin or pelvis.

Some years later I came across a follow-up study. The updated study tried to explore whether general knowledge about the body had improved over the thirty or so years since the original study.[13] The results were surprising. The study found that knowledge had not improved at all over the decades. If we just focus on the kidneys, only 27% of members of the public asked were correctly able to identify their location on an outline of the human body when offered a choice of four possible locations. This is little different from guesswork; even if everyone in the study had chosen at random, about 25% of people would still have correctly chosen the panel with the correct location of the kidneys. Maybe even more surprising was that when patients attending a kidney clinic were asked to identify the panel with the location of the kidneys, still less than half (42%) knew which of the four locations was correct.

We live in a particular cultural moment, of a democratisation of knowledge, a flattening of hierarchies and a more consumerist version of health treatments, resulting in greater individual autonomy and control. Medicine has become far more respectful of patient opinion (and again I stress that this is a good thing), and people are far more forthright about what they want, which doctors must listen to and acknowledge. However, there seems to be an ongoing disparity between what doctors and their patients understand about their bodies and their illness. Increasing access to knowledge over recent decades has not necessarily led to access to reliable knowledge. People's understanding of illness and disease, of diagnosis and of their treatments is also informed by the inevitable influences of culture, affiliations and all kinds of beliefs, in other words, by factors that really don't relate to the workings of the human body.

Expertise takes a long time to develop. As Daniel Kahneman explains in his wonderful book *Thinking, Fast and Slow*, expert intuition comes from an environment that is regular enough to be predictable and an opportunity to learn these regularities through prolonged practice.[14] I would estimate that I have spent over 20,000 patient hours in clinical psychiatry since I started practising. It has been enough time to understand what works in the short term, which is to say the immediate feedback from the consultation and the patient's response. It has also been enough time to understand the longer term: how a patient's diagnoses and treatments have stood up, and what has worked and what has not. Yet expertise has become unfashionable, as the COVID-19 pandemic showed us.

It is hard to relate now to those early days of the pandemic, characterised by uncertainty about how serious the threat of this new virus would turn out to be. It was a time of fear and confusion, and in many individuals this was followed by suspicion and mistrust. Perhaps for this reason, for a time many ordinary people fancied themselves as experts in viral transmission, coronaviruses or immunology. Having studied these things at undergraduate level, I have some notion of how complex they are, and I would not consider myself an authority. Yet I saw people with PhDs in virology being corrected by members of the public who had 'done their research'. The belief that reading a bit about something, or watching somebody talk about something, gives sufficient expertise to gainsay someone who has spent their life researching that thing, to my mind felt like a peculiarly modern concept.

The mistrust of expertise and of doctors; the suspicion of authority, governments and the pharmaceutical industry; and the contested understanding of disease and cure all found expression in the COVID-19 pandemic. It began to emerge into a movement. There was an alliance of a variety of ideologies, all of which have roots in our current culture. In some countries, the mistrust of the governing class led to an assumption that if the state recommended something, it could not be taken at face value. There was a notable reduction in uptake of the COVID-19 vaccinations amongst the black British population,[15] whose interactions with authority may not have left them with a good impression of the impartiality of the police and systems of governance. As someone whose own identity is bound up with the tragedies of the Jewish people over the years, I tried to work out how I would feel towards a semi-mandated vaccine as a Jew in tsarist Russia, or in 1930s Germany. I make no comparisons of contemporary governments to those egregious ones of the past, and I was and am fully supportive of the vaccines, but personalising the issue made it easier for me to understand what became politely known as 'vaccine hesitancy'.

The second reason for vaccine hesitancy was a more diffuse mistrust of the capitalist system. There was a narrative that pharmaceutical companies had either been complicit in the manufacture of the virus or were simply profiteering off an unnecessary and harmful vaccine. Again there was little evidence in favour of this assertion, and some solid evidence against it, not least that Astra-Zeneca were providing their vaccine on a non-profit basis during the pandemic. Yet when the facts don't fit the narrative, they are often ignored, minimised or otherwise explained away. And, not unlike the issue above with government, it cannot be denied that pharmaceutical companies have not always behaved with dignity and moral standing. One need only look at the recent opioid crisis in the US, and the role played by at least one of the pharmaceutical manufacturers there, to at least understand where the seeds of the mistrust might have been planted.

Vaccines are, by any objective measurement, one of the greatest advances in all of medicine, saving millions, perhaps billions of lives. Like any medical intervention, they will have side effects, but it is nearly always the case that for a given individual, the risk of the disease far outweighs the risk of the vaccine. The COVID-19 vaccine was perhaps the most outstanding miracle of medical ingenuity and perseverance I am likely to see in my lifetime. The media and the public were largely behind the vaccine, and pretty well all doctors. Yet what was striking was that in the biggest health crisis to have faced the world in decades, the reaction to the vaccine in many quarters was negative, based on mistrust, uncertainty and misinformation. It seemed that, for some, all the fear and anxiety and social problems caused by the lockdowns found an outlet in disagreements about the science. It was often the case that one side was informed by evidence and experience and the other was not, but somehow the debate seemed never ending.

The noisy public debate around the COVID-19 pandemic is an extreme example of a moment when the medical and scientific response to a physical illness has been widely discussed and contested. That conversation has largely died down now, as normal life has more or less resumed. The debate around the psychiatric response to mental illness may be more diffuse but it is no less challenging, not least because each generation of psychiatrists find themselves having to reassert or redefine their diagnostic boundaries anew in response to social changes. And there remains, at the margins of health and illness, a more fundamental issue of what counts as a diagnosis. Nobody would dispute that depression is a real entity, in any society and in any time period. Yet where depression blends into sadness and normal human experience is much harder to delineate. For the more culturally influenced diagnoses, the boundaries are becoming ever more blurred.

Pharmaceutical companies have obvious gains to make if more diagnoses are made. But the pressure is also coming from researchers or lobby groups advocating for their particular diagnosis or interest to be included in the diagnostic classification. And, increasingly, the push towards diagnosis is coming from patients themselves. This confluence of forces exerts considerable pressure on psychiatry, but it is important for the gatekeepers of psychiatric diagnoses to exercise care in the inclusion of new problems. The evidence for something to be considered as a diagnosis, rather than a variation of normal or a problem in someone's life, needs to be robust.

I believe in psychiatric diagnoses. I believe in them not just as a matter of professional faith, but as a thought-out and considered position. Making a diagnosis involves having a knowledge of neuroscience, psychology, sociology and pharmacology as well as human nature, in all its variety and idiosyncrasy. However, we can only really begin to take a view on the newer or more mutable diagnoses if we understand the complexity of making a diagnosis of even the more well-established and seemingly clear-cut conditions, such as dementia and schizophrenia.

4

Memories

Who are you? It is an impossible question to answer without reference to your memory: where you live, who your family and friends are, the work you do, the football team you support, the hobbies you have. This information also helps people understand and contextualise you. As you get deeper into a relationship, you will talk about where you grew up, your childhood experiences, your likes and dislikes, and the triumphs and setbacks that made you who you are. Without a memory, you would live in a world without definition, a sentient being adrift and alone. The world would be a lonely and frightening place.

Losing one's memory, the personality slowly coarsening before it gradually disappears: these are common fears. Unreliable memories are the stuff of fascination and fictional nightmares. In the futuristic film *Total Recall*, the protagonist, Douglas Quaid, decides to have an invented memory of a holiday on Mars placed into his mind so that he can enjoy the memory of being there without the expense of travelling. During the procedure, it becomes apparent that it is his current life that is a fictional memory. Suddenly he no longer knows who he is, or why this has been done to him. His job and marriage are not real, and his workmates and wife have been sent to spy on him to prevent him discovering his former, actual life. It is a chilling, disorientating and compelling concept.

Even outside of science fiction, our memories are not the stable archive of our lives that we might think. They are unreliable and subjective. The common perception, that once events are experienced they are accurately encoded in the wiring of our brain, is incorrect. We all have examples of talking to friends about a past event and each of us remembering it differently: who said what, how that person reacted and what eventually happened. All the evidence suggests that confidence in one's recollection correlates poorly with how likely that memory is to be true.

I remember once walking back home from the bus stop with my wife, Sara, soon after we got married. Halfway down the road, Sara suddenly stopped. Some fifteen metres ahead of us was a woman who had stolen money from her family years before, and had been caught buying various electronic items with their credit card. The incident had been reported to the police, and the woman had been arrested and a court date set. On the day of the trial, the woman simply failed to show up, and in the intervening years the trail had gone cold. The police found more pressing tasks to occupy them rather than chasing up minor fraudulent activity, and everyone moved on. Still, the woman was technically awaiting trial, and she was walking with a male friend only a few metres from us. We debated what to do. We briefly considered challenging her, but we had no power to detain her, and the thought of getting into a fight was not appealing.

We eventually called the police, who arrived surprisingly quickly, and here's where the trouble began. We started describing the woman and her partner, but quickly disagreed about what they were wearing and how tall they were, and when we couldn't agree on even the approximate age or race of the man accompanying her, I saw the police officer roll his eyes. I didn't blame him. We must have been pretty exasperating. It was, though, an instructive episode in how unreliable our memories can be.

This is a particular problem in criminal trials, in which eyewitness testimony can be one of the most potent pieces of evidence in a conviction. Yet eyewitness testimony, as I'd found from personal experience, can be very unreliable, and even more so after time has elapsed, when our memories decay and become distorted by a constructed recollection of what we think we saw, rather than what actually happened.

We tend to reconstruct the world from fragmentary, poorly encoded or incomplete memories in a way that usually confirms what we already believe. One 1970s study tested the memory of groups of students who were asked to read a short passage.[1] Some had their memories of what they read tested after five minutes, and others after a week. The passage was about a character, giving some facts about their life. Half the students were given a fictitious name for the character (Carol Harris), and half were told it was Helen Keller. When subjects were asked to recall what they had read afterwards, those who had been told the character was called Helen Keller 'remembered' that the original passage had talked about her being blind and deaf, just like the real-life author and activist Helen Keller, even though these conditions were not mentioned in the original passage. The same result was obtained with the fictitious name Gerald Martin and the name Adolf Hitler; subjects 'recalled' descriptions of Hitler's antisemitism, which were not included in the original passage, and did not recall reading about antisemitism when the character they had read about was called Gerald Martin. As you might expect, the results were even more stark after one week, with the distorted memories of the fictional characters becoming more pronounced as people's memories decayed. It confirmed that our memories are a reconstruction of what we think must be true as much as they are an accurate account of what actually happened. We tell ourselves a story, and fit the information into the story to make it consistent.

The Innocence Project, a US advocacy group that offers help and support to wrongfully convicted prisoners, found that of 367 cases of people who were exonerated after DNA evidence proved their innocence, 252 had been convicted based on eyewitness evidence.[2] I do not doubt that in most, if not all, cases the witnesses were entirely sincere. They would have tried their best to assist the court and ensure justice. I imagine they would have been appalled at being responsible for the wrongful conviction and prolonged imprisonment of an innocent person. In eighty-two of the cases in which DNA exonerated someone, eyewitness testimony was the *only* evidence on which the individual conviction was based. Other convictions, based on multiple eyewitness reports, revealed that *all* of the eyewitnesses were wrong. The Innocence Project website is a harrowing read. There are photographs of innocent people who have served decades in prison; lost their families, homes and livelihoods; and endured great shame and stigma before their innocence was proven. Never has the fallibility of human memory felt so poignant.

Disputed memories were all the rage when I started in psychiatry in the mid-1990s. This was a time when there was a flood of cases of what were termed 'recovered memories'. These were memories that resurfaced during therapy, most commonly with an individual claiming to remember childhood sexual abuse. Police investigations were initiated, lawsuits were begun and families were torn apart, yet the truth of an event that had often happened decades before was all but impossible to establish. The majority opinion in the scientific community was that repressed memories of abuse were unlikely. The prevailing view was that in most abuse cases the main problem was an inability to forget, rather than an inability to remember. The suspicion was that recovered memories were prompted and guided by practitioners who believed that if a patient had psychological problems, their roots must be traced back to past abuse, and it was only by unearthing these memories that a patient could make progress. One critical account of this approach, co-authored by a Pulitzer Prize-winning journalist,[3] opens by saying, 'Our goal is to prove beyond doubt that devastating mistakes are being made within certain therapy settings . . . This work is intended as an exposé of a pseudoscientific enterprise that is damaging the lives of people in need.'

The other side of the debate advanced the idea that ordinary forgetting, or defence mechanisms including repression or dissociation, concepts first developed by Sigmund Freud, could account for the memory lapses of traumatic childhood events.[4] In the case of repression, which is considered the classic Freudian defence mechanism, unpleasant memories are kept away from the conscious mind through an unconscious process to protect the individual from the distress of recalling something they would rather forget. Dissociation is a different way of avoiding emotional distress, whereby an individual acts like someone on autopilot – their unconscious mind becomes uncoupled from their conscious thought, as might happen when you arrive home after driving back on a familiar road without any recollection of the journey.

Criminal trials in which the defendant is accused of a violent offence commonly involve the defendant claiming amnesia. In murder trials, this is estimated to be in about a third of cases,[5] particularly in unplanned homicide, the so-called crimes of passion, where extreme emotion overwhelms the individual. The discovery of another lover, a blazing row and the use of alcohol or drugs are typical scenarios. These produce the kinds of heightened emotional states in which dissociation might be expected.[5] The problem is that claims of memory loss may also be used as a tactic by a violent criminal to lessen their responsibility[6] or reduce their punishment, and it is not always possible to distinguish between a ploy and a genuine case of dissociation.

For most psychiatrists, criminal trials are a world away. Complex decisions about whether someone's action was a conscious or unconscious one, or whether their amnesia for the event is real or feigned, are not something that most of us will ever normally need to think about professionally. What most of us do need to do though, and on a fairly regular basis, is decide whether memory lapses are just part of the normal everyday experience or whether they could be attributed to a psychological or neurological cause.

Complaints of memory loss are most likely to present at an outpatient clinic, as was the case with my patient Jen. The referral letter told me she was in her late forties, divorced and with grown-up children who had both emigrated. Over the past six months she had noticed her memory steadily worsening. After some investigations, including a brain scan that was returned as normal, her memory continued to decline. She had not been reassured by the routine investigations and was attending the surgery regularly, overcome with fear about what was happening.

As I walked with Jen from the waiting room, she looked on the verge of tears and panic-stricken, as if she wanted to run away. I tried to distract her with some anodyne questions – had the clinic been easy to find? How had she travelled here? Her answers, even to these benign enquiries, were fragmented, as though she was having trouble focusing, so we continued in silence until we reached my consultation room.

She seated herself at the desk across from me and unburdened herself. 'Dr Santhouse, I'm losing my mind,' she began. I was about to ask for some clarification, but the tears overwhelmed her. All the fears and anxieties she had been unable to express in the months she had been waiting for an appointment came bubbling to the surface. I waited until she was able to continue.

'It's my memory. I forget things, normal things, what I'm meant to be doing. People I've known for years, I forget their names.

Yesterday I went to the supermarket and I just couldn't remember what I'd gone for.'

I reflected on how many times I've walked into a room and stood there with my arms by my sides, wondering what I was doing there. It happens when I am overly distracted by other things in life. I've always thought I have a good memory, but most people who know me well would also consider me absent-minded, which I suppose is another word for forgetful. I forget my packed lunch, even when I've deliberately hooked it onto the door handle so that I have to walk past it on my way out. I have even tutted as I move it aside in my rush to leave the house, and only realise I've forgotten it later in the day. My life is a series of lists, without which there would be a gathering chaos of missed appointments, deadlines and other arrangements.

Now Jen was in full flow. She had developed a conviction that this was evidence of a progressive memory impairment, and these little lapses had taken on a whole new meaning. 'I'm losing my vocabulary. Like yesterday, there was a word I was trying to think of. It just wouldn't come to me. It was only on the bus on the way home that I thought of it.' She looked distraught, clutching a tissue in her right hand that she kept using to dab at her eyes or blow her nose. Her mascara was streaky now, intensifying the impression of wild-eyed panic. I passed the box of tissues along the desk back towards her, and she grabbed another.

'My whole job, my livelihood, is words,' she told me. This included previously working as a reporter for a local newspaper, and currently as a website editor. She began to fear that her deteriorating memory would mean she could no longer work. These thoughts had snowballed, so that she now feared becoming destitute and helpless – perhaps she would soon need institutional care. The thought appalled her, and she became breathless with fear as she articulated the nightmarish future she saw for herself.

Jen had been born in southern England, and she gave a detailed account of her childhood. Always a worrier, she had been diligent at school and successful in her studies, and had enjoyed playing the piano. She had studied English literature at a top university, then started to make her way in the literary world. Along the way, she fell in love, married, had two children, and then the relationship soured. Her husband had an affair with his secretary ('such a cliché', she said), whom he ended up marrying. She had been left with her two children, who had followed their own paths, leading them out of her home and into foreign lands. Now in her forties, Jen felt abandoned and destitute, with nothing but lonely and confused old age ahead.

It was striking that throughout the consultation she could give a detailed and coherent account of her difficulties. I have seen many people with dementia throughout my professional career, and nearly always they bring someone with them to give an account of their problems. The person themselves is often unaware of the myriad small ways their memory deficit is becoming apparent. They might get lost more easily when they can't create a mental map of where they are. They struggle to find common words so that their vocabulary becomes restricted. They can find it difficult to coordinate complex instructions. Following a recipe will commonly lead to chaos – timings, ingredients and measurements all require a degree of planning and forethought that few formal cognitive tests can replicate. Sometimes the dementia involves a slowing down of thinking, more an inability to retrieve memories efficiently than a loss of them, that reminds me of the ancient NHS computers using an old Microsoft operating system (they'll eventually get there with enough prompting and more time than you have to spare, but they can be slow, cumbersome and unreliable, and they are always at risk of crashing).

Jen's memory deficits did not have the feeling of a progressive cognitive decline. Her answers to questions were peppered with self-doubt and, by extension, a self-awareness commonly lacking in patients with Alzheimer's disease. Dementia can be a difficult diagnosis for a doctor. Particularly in the early stages, it can be confused with several other medical or psychiatric problems. One study found that of people referred to a memory clinic, only just over half end up with a dementia diagnosis.[7]

In many cases, as it was for Jen, an apparent failure of memory was caused not by a neurological disease but by anxiety. Part of memory involves registering new information, but when people are anxious, they are distractible; their concentration is impaired, and when people are not fully concentrating on something, it is far less likely that they will remember it.

The other aspect of memory that Jen's case highlighted is that our perception of whether our ability to retain information is normal can be related to whether we spend an abnormal amount of time thinking about it. Once we start to examine our memories or our ability to remember, it can be easy to find gaps. That's just part of life. Some things stick, others don't. Sometimes an aberration can lead to a temporary blank, such as forgetting someone's name just as you are about to introduce them (I have a terrible track record here). Problems begin with how we interpret these normal memory lapses. Things that we would have previously brushed off (forgetting names or wondering what we went upstairs for, for example) can start to take on a more sinister significance. Focusing on future potential memory lapses only amplifies the problem, until the person is convinced that they must have dementia. And that is where Jen had ended up. She was so preoccupied by what her memory lapses might signify that her life was a living torment; 'proof' was everywhere she looked, and she had all but started looking at nursing homes at the grand old age of forty-eight.

Cases like Jen's are far from uncommon. They have a name, 'functional cognitive disorders'. The word 'functional' implies that although the brain's structure is intact, so that scans show no shrinking of the brain or other signs associated with dementia, somehow the brain just isn't functioning properly. 'Functional' is intended to be a neutral term, because the function of the brain is complex and can be influenced by psychological factors. Functional cognitive disorders seem to be on the rise, and this is certainly my own experience in clinical practice. It is not clear why this is happening. One study that I came across several months after seeing Jen estimated that the proportion of new referrals attending memory services who end up with a diagnosis of a functional cognitive disorder is in the range of 12–56%.[8] I have wondered whether it is increasing exposure to an older population, often living long enough to develop dementia, that generates anxiety about memory in a younger population. Or perhaps it has something to do with fear of ageing, decline and the loss of our sense of self.

What was most interesting to me in the paper was a discussion of the factors a clinician should take notice of in a consultation that might lead to a diagnosis of a functional cognitive disorder. It included the patient giving longer answers to questions as well as being able to give a detailed account of memory failure. You might have expected that, because they suggest at least some level of intellectual function. But other factors were attending the appointment alone and bringing a handwritten list of personal problems.[8] I remember that Jen attended on her own, but had she unfurled a list of questions and worries from her coat pocket? In my imagination she did, although the details of the appointment have become hazy with time.

Similar concerns about memory can occur in post-concussion syndrome, which sometimes follows a mild head injury, the type many people have had, for example, playing sports or falling off a bike. It is an injury where there is no obvious brain damage or prolonged unconsciousness, and from a medical point of view, the person would usually be expected to recover fully. Yet in post-concussion syndrome, a person might begin to complain of concentration difficulties and memory lapses. These can be accompanied by difficulties performing mental arithmetic or other tasks requiring sustained attention. People experience persistent exhaustion, irritability, intolerance to light and noise, dizziness, headaches and poor sleep. All these symptoms start to interfere with their day-to-day activities, including work. Many patients also lose interest in their pastimes and social life, and their relationships at home frequently suffer.

Studies have shown that people are more likely to develop post-concussion syndrome if they had depression or anxiety before the head injury or are experiencing stressful life events.[9] This is not too surprising, because mental health problems usually worsen the outcome of most life events. But one of the most important factors in whether people will develop post-concussion symptoms is their attitude towards their injury. Many people with a head injury expect that it has already caused some irreparable brain damage, and continually monitor their bodies for symptoms that can be attributed to the injury.

In one study that caught my eye, the researchers asked people with no head injury to imagine they had sustained a mild head injury in a road traffic accident. They were given a list of symptoms that they might expect to develop, and interestingly the cluster of symptoms they chose was nearly identical to those seen in post-concussion syndrome.[10]

This study provided further evidence that our expectations of what is likely to occur bias us into noticing common symptoms (such as irritability, fatigue and forgetting things), which we then worry about even more, fearing that the head injury must have been more significant than we realised. This sets up a vicious cycle of anxiety, symptom focusing and the experience of symptoms. In the same study, patients who'd actually had a head injury were given the same list of symptoms and asked whether they'd had them before the head injury. They underestimated how common the symptoms of post-concussion syndrome were, which means they were far more likely to attribute normal bodily sensations like fatigue to the head injury. (As an interesting aside, the term 'immaculate concussion' was used to describe an outbreak of concussion-like symptoms amongst US embassy staff in the absence of head trauma. The problem was first observed in the US embassy in Havana, and so became known as Havana syndrome.[11])

The way in which people with post-concussion syndrome build a narrative around their symptoms, which then exacerbates them, was similar to what was happening with Jen, who had developed an anxiety disorder that was perpetuating her problems. It is easy to see how this happens: if you think that you are steadily losing your mind, anxiety seems like an appropriate reaction. In Jen's case, her anxiety was overwhelming and spread into every area of her life so that she could barely function. The hardest part of the treatment was to help her understand that, much like the post-concussion study, what she was experiencing with her memory was normal, and it was her attribution that was causing the problems. I prescribed anti-anxiety medication, and things were looking better when I saw her a month later. Once the anxiety subsided a little, she stopped thinking about and noticing her memory for brief periods, which in turn allowed her to spend more time engaged in her usual daily activities and less time thinking about her memory.

If an overanxious mind can impair memory, so too can a depressed one. In fact, depression is often behind the misdiagnosis of dementia. I've seen this plenty of times during my career. Older people with depression often appear to have cognitive impairment and behave as though their mental faculties are declining. They can be hesitant and uncertain, and complain of memory deficits. For the clinician, this can be a clue that they might not have dementia. Most people with dementia do not highlight memory deficits and will often try to conceal rather than draw attention to them. Sometimes they seem entirely and blissfully unaware of their memory problems, and many of us with relatives suffering from dementia may have wondered whether that isn't, in fact, for the best.

I remember my great-uncle's dementia. In his younger years, he was a proud, organised, disciplined man who ran a business for many years. In his later years, as dementia set in, for those who knew him well it was hard to watch. He had regressed to something more childlike. At one family dinner, he sat disengaged from the conversation, only occasionally offering a platitude or repeating a question. After the meal, as he stood up to leave, he wandered into the lounge, where there were little bowls of sweets. We watched as he tried to slide the sweets into his suit pocket, and for a moment he bore the guilty look of a schoolboy caught copying homework. We all pretended not to have noticed, but it was so sad that even decades after the event it's an image that's hard to expunge from my mind. He would have been mortified if he had developed any insight into his behaviour.

Depression appearing as dementia has intermittently reared its head in the public domain. Whilst I was at university, the Guinness trial was on the front pages of every newspaper. Four senior people at Guinness, including the chief executive Ernest Saunders, were accused and subsequently convicted of artificially raising the company's share price prior to a takeover.[12] Saunders was sentenced to prison at the age of fifty-four for a five-year term, but ten months into his sentence, at his appeal hearing, the court heard from expert witness testimony that he appeared to have early-onset dementia, which was accepted by the court and his sentence was reduced. After his release from prison, he made a recovery,[13] something so unlikely for someone with a diagnosis of early-onset dementia that three experts in old-age psychiatry wrote a letter of concern to the *BMJ*.[14] The far greater likelihood, they said, was that he had been suffering from depression, and the apparent cognitive deficits recorded were attributable to this rather than any dementia.

This case highlighted the difficulties of dementia diagnoses: that even experts can be mistaken. It also made a persuasive case for a diagnosis of Alzheimer's disease and dementia to be made using agreed diagnostic criteria to avoid getting tripped up by the many factors, such as depression, that can lead the unwary to the wrong conclusion.

I have seen many patients over the years with dementia, including from Alzheimer's disease, Parkinson's disease, multiple small blood vessel bleeds and various esoteric neurological disorders. Sometimes a mixture of pathologies causes dementia. There is the loss of brain tissue, followed by a steady decline in function and memory and a change in personality. Yet each progresses at its own pace, perhaps stressing one brain area over another, and interacting in the context of the individual, their personality and their life. It reminds me of Tolstoy's famous opening line from *Anna Karenina*, where he says that all happy families are alike, but each unhappy family is unhappy in its own way. And so with dementia, each dementia case produces its own unique tragedy.

The hardest thing of all after making the diagnosis is to say the words, to confirm the thing that everyone has been dreading. I remember Cyril, a man in his eighties who was referred to me with a change in personality. Dementia was not specifically mentioned in the referral. The personality change, it was suggested, was a consequence of the various problems arising in Cyril's life. He had endured health problems including a kind of slow-burn blood cancer, as well as the loss of his wife of over fifty years. Perhaps, the referrer speculated, the change in personality related to the difficult life events he'd had to endure and the adjustment to his new and unhappy circumstances.

Cyril attended the appointment with his son. He was wearing a navy suit, slightly baggy, and a loosely knotted tie. He looked like the retired lawyer that he was. He seemed to emanate authority, so that even in his somewhat diminished state, there were moments in the consultation where I felt cowed by his withering stare. Cyril, though, did not know why he was seeing me. Was he depressed in mood? 'Not really, no. Why?' As far as he was concerned, he could not recall any particular concerns, and in response to my probing questions, he said on more than one occasion, 'Look here, is this really all necessary?' It was accompanied by that stare, which knocked me off my stride. I kept having to explain and justify why I was asking questions, and wondering if he really didn't know, or whether this was, deep down, something so frightening to him that he did not want to face it.

His son gave a different account. Looking back, the clues had been there for a few years. His paperwork at home, normally so organised, had been piling up unsorted in various corners of the house, stuffed into shopping bags. He would start things, such as DIY, and lose interest halfway through. He was far more detached in conversations, no longer taking an active interest, and rarely initiated conversations. The son told me that his father hadn't ever seemed depressed. When I got to the more detailed cognitive testing, of memory tests and naming pictures, copying patterns and following instructions, he'd finally had enough ('Now look here ...'). I had to end the consultation. But I knew before he went for the brain scan what it was going to show. When the scan came back, you could see, unmistakably, the widened ventricles like lakes, allowing the cerebrospinal fluid to enter those areas where the brain had shrunk. Multiple dots where small blood vessels had bled, looking like drops of rain, had appeared deep in the tissues of the brain.

Alzheimer's disease is unfortunately a one-way ticket once it has taken hold. I have seen accounts of people who claim to have had dementia for decades, or say that somehow dementia is a gift, but that is not the experience of any of the many people I have met with the diagnosis. Of all the mental health problems during my nearly thirty-year career in psychiatry, the treatment of dementia must be the most disappointing. A Brazilian friend once told me of an aphorism about his homeland, as a nation that 'was, is, and always will be the country of the future'. The same could be said of treatments for Alzheimer's disease.

On the day I entered psychiatry training, a cure for Alzheimer's was only five years away. It has remained so throughout my career. The first treatments to be made commercially available, when I was a junior psychiatrist, were a class of drugs known as 'cholin-esterase inhibitors', which increased levels of a brain transmitter called acetylcholine, shown to be lower in patients with Alzheim-er's disease. The results were less than spectacular, but since it was really the only game in town, it was better than nothing. These drugs are still used and have a modest effect, but are far from the breakthrough we had hoped for.

We always believed that advances in dementia research would provide a better understanding of how the brain worked, at the detailed level of microscopic brain changes. We thought this would lead to treatments being developed based on the correction of any abnormalities. And yet I don't think there has ever been a brain disease as well understood as Alzheimer's without the treatments improving. Despite the recent euphoria around the new class of monoclonal antibody treatments, the difference they make appears modest at best.[15] I am now much closer to the end of my career than the beginning, and I'm not sure I will ever see a breakthrough treatment. But perhaps, like treatments for other illnesses such as AIDS, there won't be a breakthrough, just a series of small increments that eventually add up to a big difference.

I never saw Cyril again. After the diagnosis, his care was taken over by the older adults community psychiatry team. I was copied into the next few letters about him, which documented a gradual decline in function, until I was eventually left off the distribution list. I never saw Jen again either. She sent a note via my secretary to say that she was better and didn't need to see me any more. What had made the difference for her was relatively simple. It was in understanding the difference between normal and abnormal memory deficits, and being able to put a name to what she was experiencing. Nothing undermines people's morale more than uncertainty, nor compounds the problems that they already have. Sometimes, after the frightening limbo of facing different possible diagnoses, the simple act of giving the patient the correct one is what brings them back to themselves. It allowed Jen to take the focus away from the prison of her own fear, and once again look towards the future.

5

Schizophrenia

Some years ago, in the mid-1980s, I visited the Soviet Union. I was in my first year of university, and the idea of an adventure exploring an entirely different society and culture behind the Iron Curtain was appealing. Before I left, word had got out in the local Manchester Jewish community that I was travelling to the Soviet Union, and I was asked if I would be prepared to take some medicines and items to the refuseniks there. 'Refuseniks' was the name given to Soviet Jews who had asked to leave the country and been denied an exit visa. Asking for an exit visa was a risky business for Jews in the Soviet Union. Some would be allowed to leave; others would, entirely without reason, be denied. As a matter of government policy, the people who were made to stay, the refuseniks, were then subjected to systematic harassment and discrimination, and either assigned to the lowest-paid jobs or lost their jobs. Since it was illegal not to have a job, they would experience trouble with the police, as well as the financial difficulties that followed unemployment.

At Heathrow, I boarded an ancient Aeroflot Tupolev jet with creased carpets in the aisles and seat backs that collapsed on you if you leaned forward. The female cabin attendants were dressed in a Soviet apparatchik's impression of what Western cabin crew should wear, with cheap polyester uniforms; thick, wrinkled tights;

and heavily applied, shiny makeup. Their bored expressions were far from reassuring. Eventually the plane, after much noisy shaking and trembling, lifted off into the darkening London skies.

We touched down at Moscow's Sheremetyevo airport at 2 a.m. I quickly came to understand the difference between knowing something and experiencing something. I knew that it would be cold in Moscow in December. Yet standing at the bottom of the aeroplane steps, snow piled everywhere, with soldiers in overcoats and blue *shapkas* on their heads, stamping their feet to keep warm, I realised that until that point I had never before really felt cold. I shivered as we were driven the short distance to the terminal, where we filled out lengthy and menacing customs forms. As we stood freezing in the arrivals hall completing our forms, the tannoy crackled into life. A heavy, guttural Russian voice announced: 'No lying.' Silence. Then once again it burst into life, 'No lying.' The tannoy crackled and fell silent once more, the room now absolutely still, save for the rustling of forms being anxiously reviewed by the weary and startled passengers. I tried not to think of the tablets in my bag, which I was bringing for a refusenik with Parkinson's disease. How was I going to explain those? Luckily, I didn't have to. Finally, we were driven to the Cosmos Hotel, a forbidding state-run enterprise with a *babushka* sitting in a chair on each floor, recording the comings and goings from the rooms, which were, in any case, bugged.

I woke up the next morning with my head pounding, inches away from the radiator, the central heating being the one thing in the country, aside from the subways, that seemed to work reliably. Moscow in winter was grey and drab, the sort of city that saps the energy out of you. People on the streets walked with their heads lowered, avoiding your gaze. Everywhere were large, featureless apartment blocks, with giant posters on the sides of them proclaiming the glory of the workers. It was in one of these that I met Alexey, a refusenik on my list. He invited me into the small apartment that he shared with his large family. I remember feeling awkward at the spread laid out on the kitchen table. Just like in all the Russian books I had read, there was a samovar on the sideboard. I was doubtful they could afford such a meal, but it would have been impolite to refuse, so I sat and joined them. Alexey's English was almost perfect, and he even used English idioms. He was obviously highly educated, even if his work now was to scratch together a living doing odd jobs. Since unemployment was illegal, he was always at risk of being picked up by the police, with their pretext for arrest already in place, should he try to campaign or agitate again for an exit visa. It brought to mind something I had once heard from the former British Chief Rabbi Jonathan Sacks – that borders in democracies are there to keep people out, and in totalitarian states, to keep people in.

As we talked about the life of refuseniks like him, Alexey told me something so shocking that I wasn't sure if it had got lost in translation. He told me how the authorities would lock up political prisoners in mental institutions on the pretext of them being mentally ill. In former times, political opponents would be shot. After Stalin, the murdering of political opponents was best avoided for a country wanting to demonstrate to the world its superiority to the West. But sending people to prison could make martyrs of them, potentially creating a bigger problem. So instead, a fake diagnosis of mental illness was being used as a means of silencing political opposition. A new diagnosis was invented, 'sluggish schizophrenia', which along with 'paranoia' became a reason for involuntary detention in a psychiatric facility.[1,2]

The diagnosis could be made on any individuals whom the authorities considered fitted poorly into society. Publicly rejecting the communist ideology and political system, or political activism against the government, came under that category. Sufferers, in other words, political dissidents, might be considered to have 'reformist delusions'.[3] Whilst these character traits in any other society would be considered normal, in Soviet society, to be against the communist ideal was to invite a diagnosis of mental illness. The Soviet psychiatry theorist Andrei Snezhnevsky believed that 'patients with sluggish schizophrenia could present as ostensibly sane yet show minimal but clinically relevant personality changes that could pass unnoticed to the untrained eye'.[4] This, of course, makes 'sluggish schizophrenia' a diagnosis ripe for corruption. All the psychiatrist had to do was claim a superior, more refined perception. Symptoms of this novel form of schizophrenia included 'conflict with authorities, poor social adaptation and pessimism, and were themselves sufficient for a formal diagnosis of sluggish schizophrenia with scanty symptoms'.[4] Patients were made to take strong antipsychotic medication. They were considered cured when they no longer held views that were against the state, or at least no longer publicly expressed them. Any dissent when they left hospital would have been considered a sign of relapse, and this would be a reason to convey them to hospital for treatment once again. Sometimes, a 'patient' might be rehospitalised pre-emptively. Whenever a Western diplomat visited, for example, the 'patient' might be taken to hospital for their own good, as such circumstances were those in which relapse would most likely occur. And thus anti-Soviet demonstrations could be avoided.

In some ways, the most unpleasant part of this abuse of psychiatry was the lingering suspicion amongst family and friends that the authorities may have been justified. Whenever the former patient criticised the government, or just talked too much about the injustices of the political system, people would be inclined to wonder whether there was a touch of mental illness, after all. ('Perhaps he does seem a bit too preoccupied with the government.') The stigma of psychiatric diagnosis taints its recipients in any society.

When I discussed this political misuse of psychiatry with Dennis Ougrin, a Ukrainian colleague who grew up in the Soviet Union, I wondered to what extent the doctors involved in the process believed in the diagnoses they were giving. It seemed clear that the psychiatrists in Moscow who invented the diagnosis of sluggish schizophrenia knew what they were doing.[2] They were employed by the state for that specific purpose. But what of the psychiatrists in more remote hospitals where the patients were housed? Some of them must have realised that this diagnosis was a sham, but perhaps not all of them. There would have been some psychiatrists who accepted a diagnosis confirmed by formal state psychiatric classifications as valid. After all, diagnoses of schizophrenia and personality disorders in Western countries are all based around a shared understanding of what is 'normal'. People with personality disorders have a similar inability to function in society – they can't fit in with social norms and constructs of behaviour and struggle in the workplace and interpersonal relationships.

Consider then citizens of a country, here the Soviet Union, who jeopardise employment and relationships because of a preoccupation with an ideal: to agitate against or overthrow the government and the system that it stands for. Couldn't they be suffering from a form of mental illness? They may well be querulous, preoccupied, difficult, rigid and standing against the accepted cultural norms in their society. Perhaps they are overly suspicious about what the government is up to, and whether it might be monitoring their communications, thereby justifying the 'paranoid' part of the label. Who is to say that this personality disorder isn't a harbinger of something more serious still, schizophrenia say, even though now it may be in an early form, a 'sluggish schizophrenia'?

After my conversation with Dennis, I reflected on what my own view might have been. Would I have believed in the diagnosis of sluggish schizophrenia? Perhaps not at first, but what if the diagnosis had been around for decades and there had been conferences about it, case reports published and senior psychiatric colleagues advocating for it? There would be treatment advanced using antipsychotic medication and the newest behavioural strategies – and hey presto! The sufferer can be cured and released back into normal society. Vulnerable to relapse, of course, but at the first sign of troublesome preoccupation with the iniquities of the political system, they could always be readmitted to hospital for more effective treatment. I didn't know then, and I don't know now, what I would have done. How long would it have taken for this idea to become normalised? At what point is the diagnosis just another part of the psychiatric lexicon, uncritically accepted and left unchallenged?

Back in the land of what might be considered 'normal' psychiatry, schizophrenia is one of our less controversial diagnoses. The prevalence worldwide tends to be the same throughout different countries and across cultures, at approximately 0.3% of the population.[5] It can be reliably diagnosed, because the diagnosis has little dependence on the subjective judgements of the person making the diagnosis – the symptoms are usually obvious to any qualified psychiatrist asking the right questions. The main, although not the only, features of schizophrenia were classified by Kurt Schneider, a German psychiatrist who died in October 1967, the month I was born.[6] They are the basis for nearly all the ways schizophrenia is currently diagnosed. Auditory hallucinations are a key feature of the diagnosis. These may be noises or voices, but the sounds are not just inside your head. They are heard with crystal clarity from somewhere outside of your body, as if someone unseen really is talking to you. Sometimes the voice will be someone you recognise, although sometimes not. It can be in one or the other ear, and sometimes both. The voice may be loud or quiet, persistent or intermittent. I think it must be terrifying.

I remember once as a first-year medical student climbing the staircase to my room on the first floor of a student block. As I trotted up the stairs, I distinctly heard my name being called out. I looked around, realising with some unease that there was nobody on the staircase, either above or below me. Assuming I must have imagined it, I continued up the stairs, but when it happened a second time, with the same woman's voice clear as a bell, I froze. My heart sank. I understood in that moment what a disastrous turn my life was about to take. I remained rooted to the spot, already trying to work through the implications of a life with psychosis. It was only when I heard the voice a third time, this time located some way above me, that I looked all the way up the staircase and saw a friend leaning over the stairwell from the top floor. The relief was instant and immense. It was one of those moments that have stuck in my mind. Having very briefly experienced a fraction of the mental turmoil that someone with schizophrenia suffers, I can hardly imagine what it would be like to live with.

However, in schizophrenia the auditory hallucinations are usually far more complicated than just hearing your name. Sometimes they will be critical or derogatory comments ('you're so useless, you don't even deserve to live') and sometimes people will be talking about you in the third person ('I wonder what's got into him today?'). They can even take the form of hearing your own thoughts spoken out loud just as you think them, known by the magnificent German compound word *gedankenlautwerden*.

As an aside, one study showed how the content of auditory hallucinations has changed over the decades,[7] reflecting wider social and cultural changes. In 1930s America, hallucinations tended to be more religiously inspired and more commonly to do with behaving well (for example, hearing a voice saying 'live right'). By contrast, the psychological experiences in the 1980s indicated 'a more threatening and negative subcultural milieu'. Hallucinations had a menacing and violent tone, with commands 'to hurt' or 'to kill', and the source of the hallucinations was more likely to be attributed to the devil than an angel.[7]

The final form of hallucination in schizophrenia is hearing a running commentary on thoughts or behaviours ('He's tapping away at that keyboard. Now he's stopped again. I wonder why he keeps doing that?'). It reminds me of Jim Carrey's character in *The Truman Show*, when due to a technical hiccup he hears, through the car radio, a description of the route that he is driving and what the people around him are doing. Though the effect in real life is far more disorientating and frightening.

People experiencing this form of hallucination can end up covering windows or keyholes to take away the more obvious opportunities for people to spy on them, and when that doesn't stop the commentary, covering small holes in the room where spy cameras could be hidden. In other words, they behave like many expect people with schizophrenia to behave. As I teach my medical students, though, covering potential spyholes is, in fact, an entirely rational response if you can hear someone accurately commentating on what you are doing.

Schneider also talked about an alteration of thought possession. Most people have an intuitive sense that the thoughts they think are their own – that they originated from deep within them, even if they can't quite say how or why they started. The thoughts passing through our minds may be original or unoriginal, profound or flippant, but we understand that they belong to us and are private to us. In schizophrenia though, there is a subtle change in perception. People with schizophrenia have the feeling that thoughts in their head may not have originated with them. It feels to them as if the thoughts have simply been inserted into their head by an outside entity. Sometimes the opposite is true; they feel that their thoughts have been removed from their minds by someone. Whereas you and I may occasionally complain that we have lost our train of thought, someone with schizophrenia may see it in an entirely different and far more threatening way.

Sometimes people with schizophrenia believe that their thoughts are being projected into the minds of others, who will then know what they are thinking. It is like a form of telepathy, in which thoughts are being broadcast without trying. I remember as a medical student interviewing a middle-aged man with schizophrenia. Midway through the consultation, he stopped talking and sat bolt upright in his chair. For several long and uncomfortable moments, he maintained intense eye contact with me, before demanding that I tell him what he was thinking. I shrank into my seat, trying to reassure him that I had no such gift whilst not wanting to contradict him. The tension in the room was palpable. He became angry, tired of my denials, and my evasions only inflamed the situation until I ended up having to leave the room. It was an unnerving encounter, probably one that I would have dealt with differently with experience, recognising and reacting much sooner to the change in mood in the room. Nevertheless, it was an instructive insight into how deeply felt these seemingly unusual beliefs can be.

Paranoia is another symptom associated with schizophrenia. Those with schizophrenia commonly believe that they are at the centre of something that they are powerless to control. Years of being spied on, bugged, followed, persecuted, in danger, stalk the individual. Sufferers can be hard put to say who may be behind it all, or what is so special about them that the government or some other organisation would consider it worth spying on them.

I remember having a conversation with a woman who was convinced, after a kidney and pancreas transplant, that the hospital had inserted a microchip into her during the operation.

'What would they have done that for?' I wondered, genuinely curious.

'They want to know what I'm thinking, where I am.'

'Why? What difference would it make to them what you're doing?'

She really couldn't say. She just knew that she wanted the transplanted kidney removed, which presented a difficulty for many reasons, not least that it was highly unlikely that removing the kidney would resolve the paranoia, which would simply find another focus.

It is probably superfluous to add that the life of someone with schizophrenia is very difficult. Not only because of the awful and frightening experiences, but because social exclusion is never far behind. Employment opportunities are harder to come by. Physical health problems tend to receive less attention, because sufferers find it harder to navigate the healthcare system and follow the 'rules' of a consultation, resulting in suboptimal treatment. Families struggle to live with their affected relative. For all these reasons, schizophrenia is frequently associated with housing insecurity, unemployment, isolation and hospitalisation. It is a devastating illness, and one that seems to be definitively outside any normal experience, and yet some of the symptoms contain elements that feel somewhat relatable – in essence if not in degree.

Take paranoia, for example. At what point does healthy scepticism tip into unhealthy suspicion, and where does suspicion cross the border into paranoia? Imagine this: you walk into a bar and, as you enter, a group of people at a nearby table burst into laughter. Would it cross your mind that they may be laughing at you? Is that paranoia? It almost certainly isn't true that they are laughing at you, but which of us could honestly say that the thought would not occur to us? Do you have toilet paper stuck to your heel? Have you tucked your skirt into your knickers? Is it something about your face or your posture?

People with psychosis usually can't help referring everyday events to themselves, living in a universe in which they are at the centre, and events that happen around them are because of them. I don't think it takes much of a shift in our perception to become paranoid. How much would it take to wonder, as you walked down the street, if people were paying more attention to you than to others? How about glancing up and seeing a swivelling CCTV camera perched on its gantry, and wondering if it's following you? People who are more paranoid are not recognisably different from you and me; in fact, their way of thinking is often only a small nudge away from our own. Those things that we think of as 'other' can be far closer to us than we like to think.

What of auditory hallucinations? I've only ever had one real auditory hallucination, not the mistaken one that I described earlier. It was after a straight forty-eight hours in the hospital, back in the days when shifts of that punishing length occupied a hazy legal status. Somehow the European Union's Working Time Directive, which legally limited the working hours of all employees, exempted doctors. It was only when patients you admitted to hospital in the morning saw you on the ward that evening, and then again the following afternoon, that they would wonder aloud if you ever went home. I often wondered the same thing myself. (The second thing patients wondered, reasonably enough, was whether it was safe for you to treat them.) On this occasion, I had arrived home at about 10 a.m., and as soon as I got home, I slipped off my shoes and sat on the couch, thinking about having breakfast. Some time later I was awoken by the sound of school-children laughing and chattering in the excitable and energised way that they do. As I regained consciousness, I could hear them outside the window, the sound starting to fade. By now I couldn't understand why they had come down my street, since there was no school nearby and my road was not particularly on the way to anywhere. I walked to the window at the front of the house to be met by a picture of quiet residential suburbia. The postman was at the far end of the street, there were a couple of people with shopping bags, but the children were an illusion. My first hallucination was a bewildering and unsettling experience.

I had experienced what is called a hypnopompic hallucination – those hallucinations that occur on waking from sleep (the opposite, hallucinations that occur on falling off to sleep, are known as hypnagogic). They can be auditory, as mine was, or visual (many years later I had one of these too, a spectral figure of a Tudor woman in a red dress and hat hovering near my bed as I awoke in the night – the only time in my life I have ever screamed in fear).

Hypnagogic and hypnopompic hallucinations are most famously associated with the sleep disorder narcolepsy, in which people have sudden and irresistible urges to sleep at inappropriate times. Yet one study in the *British Journal of Psychiatry* looked at how common these types of auditory hallucinations were in the general population.[8] The results were surprising. Of almost 5,000 individuals chosen as representative of the general population, 37% reported hypnagogic hallucinations and 12.5% hypnopompic hallucinations. In other words, these brief hallucinations are actually quite common. Persistent auditory hallucinations are far less common and much more suggestive that something serious has gone awry.

Yet even if the hallucinations associated with schizophrenia and other serious mental illnesses are more persistent, the way that they are interpreted varies across different cultures. In Western cultures, the quickest shorthand to ask if someone is mentally ill – and the fastest way to give offence – is to ask if they hear voices. We imbue this with such a significance that over the years I have learned to tiptoe towards this symptom with a series of innocuous-sounding questions to avoid an indignant reply of 'I'm not mad, doctor!' I usually start with something suitably vague like, 'During times of stress (and absolutely everybody thinks they are under stress), people often report having unusual experiences. Has anything like that happened to you?' Some people will then unburden themselves of their hallucinatory experiences, but for those unsure of what I mean, I go on to say that people report hearing noises – or possibly voices – when there doesn't seem to be anyone around. I have learned to phrase it in a way that is depersonalised, normalised, all attributable to 'stress', so that the person can admit to these experiences without feeling they are admitting to something 'mental'. Contrast this with other cultures, in which auditory hallucinations may be seen as attempts from the spirit world to contact them,[9] or possibly trying to possess them, but not necessarily as harbingers of mental illness. What passes as pathological in one culture can be seen as far more acceptable, even normal, in another.

I saw Lloyd some years ago, in one of his first hospital admissions. He was in his late teens, just out of school and still living with his parents. Things had started to go wrong a few months before the time we met. It started with Lloyd's increasing preoccupation with religion and the devil. There was no background of religious adherence in the family, no real point of reference for the family to make sense of what was going on for him. Initially, this new interest seemed quite benign to his parents, like a young man trying to work out his values in life. Lloyd himself told me that problems began when YouTube videos about religion kept popping up in his feed. He knew this could not be a chance occurrence and quickly understood it as a sign that he needed to engage in the fight against the devil. He came to believe that the eternal battle between the forces of light and darkness was taking place and he was caught in the middle. It was all-consuming, and he was terrified. He believed that people in other houses knew what he was thinking ('How do you know?' I asked him. 'I just know.') and that his thoughts were being projected outwards to them by means that he could not even guess at. He was sure that his friends were talking about him, and initially challenged them, and then at some point gave up and withdrew from social contact. He feared his food may be poisoned. Sometimes he heard voices speaking about him, auditory hallucinations that seemed to come on when there were noises in the pipes at home. He didn't know if he could take it any more.

He had been in hospital for around two weeks when I next saw him, and he had been taking antipsychotic medication. Although his symptoms were still present, they lacked their previous intensity and carried less emotional resonance. He was starting to develop some insight into his mental experiences. He no longer minded taking the medication, although he did not like the side effects, particularly the dry mouth. He lit up a cigarette as we spoke. Smoking was still allowed back then on the wards – and nearly every inpatient seemed to do it. He had only started smoking since coming to the ward. 'It's a bad idea,' I told him. 'Not good for you. I'm going to tell your mother.' He looked up, startled and guilty, like the schoolboy that he had recently been, and we both laughed. But the levity was just superficial. Underneath it was the understanding that he was a young man embarking on his journey in life under some of the most difficult circumstances, with an inpatient psychiatric admission before his twentieth birthday, and his future far from certain.

I thought back to his initial presentation, which began with such religious fervour. Perhaps in former times in England, he would have been revered as having special powers or insights. In other cultures, his symptoms may have had an entirely different meaning. But ultimately, if you put enough symptoms of psychosis together, even if they include religious fervour, or hearing voices of angels speaking to you, here in England in the twenty-first century at least, schizophrenia is likely to be considered as a diagnosis.

Psychiatry is a discipline that predominantly developed in the West, and the diagnostic guidelines developed for illnesses like schizophrenia are based primarily on Western belief systems. One fascinating study looked at the way the Iban people of Malaysia understood the standardised Western questionnaires trying to elicit schizophrenia symptoms.[10] Whilst we take it as axiomatic that our thoughts originate from somewhere within our brains, for the Iban, thoughts or emotions can arise from the heart. As the authors of the study go on to say, in Western cultures we understand personhood as 'a mental life that is recognised as being located in the brain'. For the Iban, the notion of personhood is defined 'more in terms of the interactions with those that surround him or her'.[10] This is a less individualised concept of personhood than we have in the West, and personhood is not seen as a reflection of the individual's mental experience. This means that when questionnaires translated into the local language ask about thoughts being inserted or removed into people's heads, or broadcast to others, the Iban framework for thinking about who they are is so different to ours that the questions simply don't make sense.

I have often wondered how we would feel if the situation were reversed. Suppose someone inhabiting another culture,[11] one with an entirely different belief system such as a traditional African culture, were to visit us to study our mental health. Let's suppose we have been experiencing some mental struggles, and the researcher, working through their checklist, asks if we have experienced these symptoms because our ancestors are angry with us. Next, they ask if our illness may have resulted from something we had done to offend the spirit world. We would have no frame of reference to answer these questions, no real way of relating to them. We would feel that they hadn't really 'got' us. Their models of explaining illness would be seen as irrelevant, unhelpful, perhaps annoying. We may try to be helpful to the researcher, explaining that we had been under significant stress, dealing with overwhelming and competing demands on our time and suggesting that, in our opinion, this combination of pressures had led us to this crisis. The researcher would look at you, frowning, pen hovering over the clipboard, pressing you to answer the questions.

After years of being trained in one belief system, and even just after growing up surrounded by certain cultural beliefs, it can be easy to become blind to the frame of reference we use to explain certain symptoms. Often, what we think of as normal appears so self-evidently true that we don't even consider challenging it. Yet parts of the world do not share our views of what is normal, even in an area as deeply researched as schizophrenia.

One of the first things I learned about the treatment of schizophrenia is that despite our access to newer and more sophisticated drug treatments, the outcomes in Western countries are not necessarily better than those in developing countries. In fact, more than one analysis has suggested that low- and middle-income countries do better than the West for schizophrenia outcomes.[12] There has been much speculation about why this might be. I believe the answer is related to the framework through which we view abnormal mental experiences and interact with those people experiencing them.

When I first started at the Maudsley Hospital in 1996, one of the only professors I knew was Julian Leff, because he was the father of one of my closest friends, Alex, himself now a professor of neurology. Julian was known in the hospital for his shock of curly white hair and his summer safari suits. In the wider world, he was famous for his research, particularly his interest in the social factors influencing outcomes in schizophrenia, something that he continued to develop even when other researchers were moving into the more 'biological' areas of psychiatry.

His most celebrated research was on what was called 'expressed emotion'.[13] Expressed emotion describes those families where there is a large amount of critical comment directed at the individual with schizophrenia. He and his colleagues showed that individuals with schizophrenia who were discharged from hospital to a family with high expressed emotion had a high rate of relapse. Nine months after discharge, 48% of them were found to have relapsed. For those returning to an environment of low expressed emotion, only 6% had relapsed.[13] At two years after discharge, an environment with low expressed emotion was even more important than medication in preventing relapse of schizophrenia.

This research finding has remained robust, yet in the UK it is hard to find people practising family therapy in the community to actively reduce expressed emotion. Even when I was still a trainee, social psychiatry was on a downward trajectory, and instead the focus was on more targeted antipsychotic medications and MRI scanners that showed real-time brain activity. Julian Leff would visit community mental health teams and give advice on how best to manage family dynamics and reduce expressed emotion, but he seemed to be a lone voice.

For all the emphasis we have placed on medical treatments since I qualified, the outcomes of schizophrenia would benefit from measures that, elsewhere in the world, seem to be more common. Social inclusion of people with schizophrenia, less judgement of them, and an acceptance within homes and communities would likely all be protective against relapse.

The rates of schizophrenia worldwide are remarkably similar. It is probably one of the most robust of the psychiatric diagnoses. Yet even in this area of psychiatry, where diagnosis is relatively uncontroversial, there can still be debates about where the boundaries of normal lie. How these mental experiences are understood in a particular culture can influence whether or not they are seen as mental pathology. And the flip side is true too. Normal human experience and dissent can be pathologised by those unscrupulous enough to want to do so. Such cases tend to be the exceptions though.

For other diagnoses, where the variation from normal can involve more of a subjective judgement, where the symptoms of illness are obvious at one end but can blend into those experienced by most people at the other end, the dangers of misdiagnosis are far greater. For these, we need to be even more careful about defining where the borders are between normal and abnormal mental health.

6

The Evolution of Depression

Sian had come to see me because she felt depressed. She couldn't remember how many psychiatrists and therapists she may have seen before me. We were about halfway through the consultation when the question came up. There was a pause.

'Well, it must have been . . . I mean, do I include counsellors at school?'

I nodded. Why not?

'Well,' she began again, and started counting on her fingers, then ran out of them and said, 'at least ten'.

I wondered if I should get a chronology, but the passage of time often makes a chronology unreliable, so I thought it would be easier to start with a summary. After more counting on her fingers, she told me she had seen at least three counsellors, three psychologists, two psychotherapists and four different psychiatrists she could remember, over the course of twenty years. She was now in her mid-thirties, so she must have been in therapy of one sort or another all of her adult life, as well as for a large part of her childhood.

I wondered why she still had any confidence in the medical profession. Here she was, some two decades after her first interactions with mental health services, and really was she any better?

I considered what I had to offer, over and above what had been offered before. There is vanity in most of us; we like to think that we may be the psychiatrist or therapist to succeed where others have failed. I have heard it called a rescue fantasy, or a hero complex, and either way it doesn't sound very healthy. But if I'm really honest with myself, I'm not immune to it. I wanted to be the person who made her better.

I thought back to when I was a psychiatry trainee. My boss at the time was being flattered by a patient. She told him that nobody had been able to cure her. With his reputation and expertise though, she knew he would be able to help. There was a pause as he considered his reply. It was the opportunity for him to modestly declare that he couldn't, of course, admit to his superior reputation but would do his very best.

'It's been my experience,' he said eventually, 'that usually where other people have failed, then so will I.'

I remember being taken aback. I thought his response was ungenerous and negative. Why not let the patient have hope? Yet over the years, I have come round to his point of view. It's not a good idea to be guided by your vanity. Being positive and optimistic is generally helpful, but allowing yourself the quick hit of feeling superior to the clinicians who have preceded you and failed usually doesn't end well. It's always better to underpromise and overdeliver in such situations.

Sian's problem, the one that had been going on for all these years, was that she was unhappy. For as long as she could remember, nothing had given her much pleasure. She just didn't seem to enjoy life as she knew other people did. Nothing had gone dramatically wrong for her, nothing she could point to as the root cause of all her trouble, and this somehow made it worse.

She had grown up in a fairly normal household. Her father had been a university lecturer and her mother was once a librarian, although she stopped working when Sian was born. There was enough money to provide for her material needs, although she described her parents as 'a bit on the spectrum' and thought that her emotional needs were less readily attended to. She was academically above average, but hadn't much cared for school and wasn't entertained by the classroom pranks. She liked to play netball and made a few friends, but tended to spend time on her own. Because she lived near the sea, she took up surfing, which was her main hobby.

As we spoke, I observed that she did not have an easy manner. More than that, she seemed to generate a pall of negativity around her. She told me she had tried cutting herself on a few occasions in her teens, some scratching on her forearms with scissors, but discovered that it hurt without providing any cathartic relief, and soon stopped it. Over the years, I had learned not to overreact to this kind of admission – especially if the patient had tried it only once or twice. Self-harm had become something of a phenomenon over the last two decades. A study in Ireland showed an increase in self-harm of 22% from 2007 to 2016, with the biggest increase in ten- to fourteen-year-olds.[1] It often seemed to happen in clusters in schools, and I had seen a lot of it in my clinics. I don't recall a single incident during my own school days. Distress wasn't invented in the 2000s, but somehow this particular response to dealing with it seemed to have found this new and upsetting form.

Sian summed up her childhood in one word: 'alone'. It was a feeling that persisted through university, where she studied economics, and into her adult life. She had taken a job with a bank, where she was making reasonable money, and had recently bought her own one-bedroom flat. She had embarked on a new relationship two months previously, and although it was a relatively recent one, she spoke of it with little enthusiasm. He hadn't been in her life, and now he was. I sensed that soon he wouldn't be again. Nothing seemed to give her pleasure. She still didn't have many friends, and although she felt loyalty and a connection to her family, this wasn't expressed in regular contact or great warmth. She told me that everyone around her was happier than her, somehow normal, whereas she described her own life as just 'drifting along'.

As she spoke, I began to see things from her point of view. I could understand that, if you don't have the capacity to feel much pleasure, then life must seem like a lengthy and joyless ordeal, something to be endured rather than savoured. Sometimes it can be hard not to get drawn into the patient's perspective. Whilst understanding another's point of view is referred to as empathy, and is seen as a good thing, the downside is that it can stifle your thinking, and you can soon start to feel the same waves of hopelessness and futility as your patient.

I wondered how she knew how happy other people were. What was her reference point? How did she know that other people were always happier than her? I imagine we have some intuitive sense of it, but it's surely hard to tell. If you look around at strangers on the tube, or even at your friends, people are rarely obviously 'happy'. They have life's problems and challenges to overcome. There are heating bills, food prices, inflation, sick relatives, mean bosses, poor employers, bereavements, failing relationships. There are misbehaving children, illnesses, delayed trains, traffic jams, never-ending emails, renewals of insurance policies, expensive car maintenance, vehicle breakdowns, road traffic collisions, difficult neighbours, incompetent leadership, pointless wars, leaking roofs, credit card bills, unjust accusations, failing businesses, cheating partners, climate change, and probably many more. How happy are we meant to be?

Depression is meant to be different in kind rather than in degree from normal. We don't talk about being 'on the spectrum' for depression. But then how should we think about a case like Sian? She had carried a persistent feeling of discontent with her life, a sense of joylessness from her daily existence, for as long as she could remember, that never quite developed or receded. At what point does a normal level of unhappiness tip over into depression?

Depression has been recognised since biblical times, when it was recorded that David played a harp to relieve King Saul of his melancholy. Later, Hippocrates theorised that melancholia was caused by an excess of black bile, an imbalance in the normally well-regulated four 'humours' within the body. For centuries after that, theories of depression were largely based around Hippocrates' humoural theory, until the seventeenth century. After this time, theories about the causes of depression developed, moving on to the nervous system, to psychodynamic theory and then to the brain and neurochemistry.[2] Modern psychiatry would frame depression as a classic bio-psycho-social illness. Starting with the biological, for some there is a genetic susceptibility to the illness, perhaps underlying the changes in brain chemistry and function seen in depression. These alone may not be enough to trigger the symptoms. The onset (and maintenance) appears to be influenced by social adversity as well as psychological factors, of how the world and events are interpreted around us, and our perceived ability to manage or control them.

Depression, like all psychiatric diagnoses, is defined by its symptoms. There is no objective measure, no yardstick, no blood test that will give a definitive answer, and therein lies the problem. When it is severe, depression really couldn't be mistaken for anything else. People with severe depression are withdrawn, sometimes to the point of being mute, their anguish etched onto their face. I have seen people so depressed that they have become catatonic, a state whereby they sit inert, not attempting to eat or drink, simply staring ahead into the unfathomable blackness of their despair. I have seen other patients with psychosis accompanying their depression. They have hallucinations, hearing voices confirming, in the most direct and critical way, the patient's worthlessness. In one case I saw, the patient was convinced he smelled of rotting meat, could feel it in his nostrils and was repulsed by it. He was sure everyone else could smell it too – passengers on buses that he took, shopkeepers in local stores – and were disgusted by him.

Such cases of severe depression are uncommon and hard to forget. Most cases of depression don't look like this though, which is not to say they are mild. Even moderate depression can still have a range of deeply unpleasant and disabling symptoms. Depression is not just sadness but an inability to take pleasure from the things that the individual used to do. Life is greyer, less appealing. Individuals are suffused with a sense of pessimism and pointlessness. There is commonly a feeling of helplessness, a belief that nothing they could do is ever likely to alleviate their cares, often to the extent that they just stop trying. Such thoughts can lead to suicidal thinking, and sometimes suicidal acts. Most patients I see with symptoms like this are barely functioning in their normal lives. Work is a struggle, if not impossible, and they have withdrawn from social and other activities.

Yet in the milder types of depression, symptoms can be relatively sparse and merge into experiences that many of us could identify with. Who can honestly say that they have never experienced sadness, low mood, loss of enthusiasm, poor sleep, despair, loss of appetite? – all of which are scorable symptoms of depression. In Sian's case, this had also included persistent feelings of discontent with her life, a sense of joylessness from her daily existence, for as long as she could remember, that never quite developed or receded. Her symptoms added up to what has been described as dysthymia, a persistent state of low mood whereby individuals just seem to spend life bumping along the bottom. Antidepressants commonly don't help, and there's not much evidence for the effectiveness of talking therapies. Dysthymia has been the subject of debate as to whether it is related to depression or whether it should best be considered a personality variant,[3] in the way that some people are born optimists and others, by dint of their nature, tend towards negativity and hopelessness.

Either way, there are now many more people attending their doctors with low mood, and a significant increase in the number of cases of depression being diagnosed. In the US, studies report that the proportion of people who have had depression in the past year has increased over the course of this century. In 2005, 6.6% of the population had experienced depression within the past year, which had risen to 7.3% in 2015, 8.6% in 2019 and 9.2% in 2020.[4] They are staggering figures, considering the numbers of people these percentages represent. What might be causing this increase?

There has long been evidence that social factors may lead to or create a vulnerability to depression. The classic study about social factors was from the 1970s, which looked at depression in women, one of those studies that has become iconic in the world of psychiatry, although its findings may seem self-evident now.[5] The authors showed that women were more likely to become depressed if they had no occupation outside the home, as well as more than three children at home under the age of fourteen. Loss of their own mother in childhood and lack of a confiding relationship also compounded the risk. The commonality of all of these factors is social isolation. This is easy to identify with. Whenever I had to look after my four young boys on my own for a weekend, going back to work on Monday morning was the finish line that I aimed at. Wonderful and loving though the boys were, the work of looking after them was demanding and relentless, and having to face that on my own over months and years without variation in the routine or someone to share the experience with would have been more than I could have withstood.

What is it in the social environment today that may account for the increased rates of depression? Compared with the conditions of the Victorian working class, or the serfs working the land in the Middle Ages, our era is one of unparalleled luxury in most Western nations. There is poverty in our society, but it is more commonly poverty relative to those who have more, rather than absolute poverty where people have no shoes, food or shelter.

And yet, alongside the material gains, we have lost a sense of social cohesion. In times gone by, it would have been all but impossible to exist alone. Now it is possible to survive outside of a community, and many people are disconnected from the society around them, even having the majority of their interactions through a screen. Those interactions that give people a sense of mattering, of being part of something bigger than themselves, can get easily lost. The resulting loneliness and disconnectedness are potent causes of misery. It was no surprise that one of the most significant effects of the COVID-19 lockdowns was a rise in cases of depression and anxiety.

I would add two further points here. The first is that we live in a society where people's worth is measured by their productivity. Those who struggle to be productive can quickly come to the view that there must be something deficient within them. In a broadly capitalist system, which most liberal democracies tend to be, value judgements are quickly made of another's worth based on parameters that really shouldn't matter. In early modern England, social hierarchy was divinely ordained,[6] and whilst suffering may have been prevalent, the sense of shame and failure may not have been. It seems that, contrary to our modern view of things, acceptance of difference in earlier societies was better than we might have thought. There is some evidence that those with physical disabilities were treated well in prehistoric societies, essentially accorded the same dignity as the rest of society.[7] This can be seen in the bone mineral densities at burial sites, where people with disabilities were comparable to their able-bodied peers, suggesting that they had received similar nutrition. It can be seen in the respect with which they were buried, for example, with tools and the usual burial paraphernalia. One historian argues that in past centuries, people with disabilities may have enjoyed more rights than they do today.[8] Jobs were found wherever possible for people to work at their own pace, thereby gaining respect – and self-respect – rather than the marginalisation that can happen in more modern societies.

The second point relates to religion. For much of society's history, the population took religion seriously. Religion was ever-present in people's lives; it made sense of their suffering, the punishment here on earth offsetting some of that in the afterlife. People's expectation of life was of an eternal struggle. Likely their friends and neighbours were enduring the same, and they were all undergoing hardships with the expectation of a better afterlife. Maybe suffering now has come to be seen as meaningless. It offers no cathartic role, nothing that elevates the spirit on its journey to the afterlife. Meaningless suffering, as Holocaust survivor Viktor Frankl said, is what breaks the spirit and makes life intolerable.[9] Language and vocabulary change, and expectations of what our lives should be have changed. Would Sian have seen herself as 'ill' in the Middle Ages? It's a difficult question to answer. I understood that life was hard for her to navigate. Nobody sits in front of a psychiatrist for want of something more entertaining to do. People come to a psychiatrist because they are suffering and believe the best way to conceptualise their suffering is as a mental illness. But to what extent does the language we have help us frame our problems and make sense of them in our current cultural context of illness and health?

Perhaps part of the explanation for the rise in depression lies in people's greater comfort in admitting to having a lower mood and seeing their doctor. It can be hard to remember that it was only a generation ago that depression for many people was seen as something to hide, perhaps even from yourself. Men particularly have been reluctant to seek help for depression, often attending their doctor with a physical complaint, hoping that the doctor will work out they are depressed, and not mentioning it if the doctor doesn't. To counter some of these engrained attitudes, the Royal College of Psychiatrists ran a 'Defeat Depression' campaign from 1992 to 1996, an attempt to change the public view of depression.[10] The campaign was fairly successful in reducing stigma and changing attitudes to treatment, increasing the acceptability of antidepressant medication, and I viewed the campaign both then and now as a good thing. And yet, there is a question over whether this increasing awareness of depression has altered what we think of as depression and how we view our own experiences.

In the wake of the campaign, a survey asked people if either they, a family member or a close friend had experienced depression. Around 25% of respondents thought they had experienced depression, and 32% thought a close family member probably had.[10] I wondered whether, if I had been at university now, I would have qualified for a diagnosis of depression. The life of a medical student could be isolating. There were always exams to pass and essays to write, and we always seemed to have a heavier workload than students of other subjects. There were days on end when I sat on my own, listening to The Smiths and feeling friendless, sad and lacking in all drive and energy. I remember one day, sitting on a bench next to a river after a week or two like this, reading a university pamphlet on 'the blues' and relating to all of it. If a student today had those symptoms, I am pretty sure they would receive a diagnosis and be prescribed treatment. Yet at the time I never considered it. I was sad, lonely, demotivated, fed up and once or twice on the point of tears, but back then depression felt to me like another country.

I'm not sure what I expected my life to be, or how happy I thought I would be. I somehow developed the subconscious idea, a reflection of my own upbringing and generation, that the world of work was one of joyless self-sacrifice. I watched my father leave and return from a place of work that he never really spoke about with enthusiasm. He just went in the morning and came back in the evening. He was often stressed and anxious, a family trait, but not unhappy. He reminded me of the dad in Judith Kerr's *The Tiger Who Came to Tea*. Work–life balance, fulfilment, happiness, job satisfaction were all alien concepts yet to be invented, or at least talked about. It's different now. The language has changed, along with expectations. There has been a trend over recent years for people to describe themselves as 'passionate about' teaching, com-mittee work, pensions or whatever work they do, and it always makes me feel terrible. I have enjoyed my job well enough, and reading gives me pleasure, but passionate? I thought that word was reserved for the first fortnight of a new relationship, not the sustained grind of a career. Perhaps I was doing it all wrong, or maybe I wasn't feeling what I was supposed to be feeling. In truth, I'm pretty sure it is a fiction, in the way that 'thriving under pressure' is a fiction. Nobody thrives by feeling sick when they wake up in the morning, and what people probably mean is that they don't mind being busy. But the words and phrases that become commonplace can start to make others wonder whether they are feeling about life what they are supposed to. If you think that other people are happier than you, experiencing that giddy rush of joy on their commute to work, does that mean you are depressed?

It comes back to the boundaries of depression, and whether thinking you have got depression and you actually having it are the same thing. Working in a general hospital for many years, I attended regular meetings with surgeons and physicians, as well as the wider multidisciplinary team of nurses, physios and occupational therapists, to discuss our joint patients. At one meeting, about a complex patient with depression who needed a kidney transplant, one of the doctors jokingly said to me that I had the far easier job, because patients would just tell me their diagnosis. Like many jokes though, it seemed to say something that I imagine he, like many people, thought was true. It is a popular misconception that an individual declaring themselves depressed should be considered to have depression. Maybe, and maybe not. But what it illustrates is that we have come to think of depression as a list of symptoms in a classification system, or perhaps just little more than someone saying that they feel depressed or sad.

In a paper, the US psychiatrist Kenneth Kendler[11] looked back at how depression was described in the medical literature during the first half of the twentieth century. He showed that earlier authors used a variety of terms such as 'broken hearted' or 'in agony' or 'wretched'. There were some symptoms that almost all psychiatrists of that earlier period considered central to the diagnosis of depression, such as speech that is 'slow, hesitant, indistinct and/or monosyllabic', or anxiety and depersonalisation (a sense of disconnectedness, as though you, or the world around you, are not quite real) that don't appear at all in today's DSM – although they are present in nearly all the cases of significant depression I have seen. In fact, many people, including psychiatrists, no longer consider that depersonalisation is a feature of depression. Today, the richness of those past descriptions of depression has given way to DSM's definition as feeling 'sad' or 'empty' and a checklist of symptoms.

But is a checklist of symptoms the best way of making a diagnosis? As Kendler said, we have taken the index of a thing for the thing itself.[11] What he meant was that we have started to confuse a list of symptoms for the actual illness. The classification systems we use to diagnose things like depression are there to make sure of a certain orderliness to the diagnosis. They increase reliability, which is to say that different people in different healthcare systems should reach the same conclusion about the same patient by ticking off a list of symptoms that a patient should meet. But Kendler's point was that this list of symptoms is not the disease itself. An analogy might be that a blob on a chest X-ray is not necessarily lung cancer. It may look like cancer, but it isn't the cancer itself. The cancer is some cells that are dividing in an uncontrolled way in the chest. The X-ray is a piece of evidence that might suggest cancer as a diagnosis, but it could in fact be an infection, haemorrhage or inflammatory disease, amongst many other diagnoses. A course of chemotherapy would never be given based on a suspicious X-ray finding alone.

Similarly, in psychiatry the checklist of symptoms is effectively the X-ray rather than the illness. Making a diagnosis of depression is a separate and more thoughtful process. Working out the best way of treating a patient's depression requires equal care and judgement. Yet somehow, as the delivery of psychiatry has become more pressured and as people labour under the misapprehension that doing it must be easy because the patient simply tells you the diagnosis, we are going to keep seeing the expansion of diagnoses. Doing psychiatry well takes time, a commodity in short supply in most clinic appointments.

Depression is one of the commonest mental illnesses and therefore one of the most frequent referrals to a psychiatrist. It is easy to manage badly, and you can do so without attracting any criticism. Simply go through a checklist of symptoms of major depressive disorder, count them off and prescribe an antidepressant if the number of symptoms exceeds the threshold. This is what had happened with my patient Elena. When she came to see me, she was on a cocktail of four different antidepressants. She explained that she had been on antidepressants throughout her teenage years in Romania. She was now in her early twenties and had come to London as a data engineer for a large multinational company. She was looking for a psychiatrist in London to continue prescribing her medicines and had noticed that I worked conveniently close to her accommodation. It was hardly a ringing endorsement, either of me or of her belief in the possibility of her improving.

We spent the first consultation, an hour, taking a history. We spoke of her symptoms, upbringing, life and relationships. There was ten years of narrative to unravel concerning the depression itself, and by the end of the consultation I concluded that a diagnosis of depression was probably correct, but I still wasn't entirely clear how she had ended up on so much medication. Usually, a single antidepressant is sufficient, occasionally two are needed if depression is proving hard to treat, but four? It is almost unheard of. It suggested to me either a serious depression that is not responding to all the usual treatments or, more likely, unconventional prescribing. I told her that the first thing we needed to do was cut back the antidepressant treatment and use a single medicine at a proper therapeutic dose. Elena was a thoughtful woman, and she thought about what I said, before politely rejecting it. In retrospect, I shouldn't have been so fast to undermine her current treatment plan.

The next time we met, we got into a discussion about our previous appointment. What had struck her, she said, was how I didn't use any rating scales to measure her mood. Elena said that this was how nearly all of her previous appointments had gone. A chat with the doctor, the completion of some rating scales and an action based on the results of these, usually a change related to antidepressant prescribing. What it came down to was that she didn't really trust me. She trusted the rating scales, an objective measurement, a number that reflected her mood. Except, as I tried to point out, rating scales are not necessarily measuring something real. You can measure fatigue, appetite, concentration and restless-ness, and all of these can be scored highly without the individual being particularly depressed, even though they are all potentially symptoms of depression. I explained that I am not against rating scales, and they do have a place in providing an objective measure of treatment progress, but they are of little value in making a diag-nosis in comparison with engaging with and trying to understand the patient in front of you.

It took some time for Elena and I to align on her treatment plan, because it took me some time to realise we had different under-standings of what might constitute effective treatment. There was her belief, implied but never stated, that more medicine is better medicine, and she was happy being on four antidepressants. This is more prevalent in some cultures than others, and I see it in many patients from the US, as well as some from Eastern Europe. In the US it led to the 'Choosing Wisely' campaign, an attempt to curb the waste and excess in US healthcare, with a figure of 30% quoted for the proportion of expenditure in healthcare wasted.[12] The UK is not immune from wasteful healthcare spending, of course, and we have had our own 'Too Much Medicine' campaign to try to reduce this. But we are not, by and large, incentivised to prescribe particular medications, and thankfully we are spared the direct-to-consumer advertising, which is legal in the US, that adds additional pressure from patients to prescribe particular medications.

Eventually, we agreed to prescribe just one medication at a therapeutic dose. It was gratifying to see that she soon recovered to the point that she no longer reported any symptoms of depression, although this meant her remaining on the single antidepressant to have a further period of stability. Depression is vulnerable to relapse in the months after recovery, and continued antidepressant use can reduce this risk. But since she was back to normal, I was able to discharge her from the clinic, with a flurry of gratitude from her that cheered me up for the rest of the day. Yet her case highlighted the reliance on rating scales and ever-increasing medication treatments. It seemed to reflect a certain commodification of depression, as though you could see a dozen cases quickly using this method. It made me think of a prototype AI psychiatrist.

It is hard to blame doctors working under pressure. It is understandable to use a kind of shortcut to diagnosis in the context of limited time and an urge to do something for the patient in the room, but it often means that antidepressants are given to people with all sorts of problems that are not depression at all, even if they share some of its features. Made badly, a diagnosis of depression obfuscates and hides complexity, distilling problems down to a single word. Antidepressants cannot treat the weight of the twenty-first century and its inequities, nor can they treat thwarted ambition or messy and unfulfilled lives. Perhaps it is the diagnosis the patient is expecting, but antidepressants are often not the answer.

I remember seeing Ron in an outpatient clinic one October morning. The referral seemed straightforward enough. It was in the form of a letter from his GP asking for an assessment of a depressive illness. Ron was in the waiting room, a man in his twenties, looking surprisingly chirpy. He was reading a book, with a paper cup of coffee on the little table next to him, as though he was settling down for a long wait. The book he was reading was one that I had recently read and had loved, so we talked about *A Gentleman in Moscow* on the way to the consultation room, laughing at the absurdity of the main character's situation: confined to an expensive hotel in Soviet Russia because the revolutionaries wanted to kill him for being an aristocrat, but couldn't because they mistakenly thought he'd written a revolutionary poem.

After we sat down, we got down to the main issue at hand. We talked about Ron's mood, as well as the onset and progress of the depression that he had come for advice about. It was hard to make a case for Ron being currently depressed. His lively conversation about the book on the way from the waiting room was a reflection of the way he had been feeling over the preceding months, which was generally upbeat and positive. As a consultation, it felt odd. It is unusual for people to be well when they come to my outpatient clinic for the first time. But Ron's issue was not that he was depressed, but that he anticipated becoming depressed soon. As the days grew shorter, he felt sure that his seasonal affective disorder (SAD) would return. He wanted me to write a prescription for antidepressants that he could start to take in November.

His concern was understandable. He was worried that depression might affect his ability to work. He had been writing features in a lifestyle magazine for the past eighteen months, which was the first stable employment he had ever had. It was a job that aligned with the ambitions he had carried since leaving college six years previously. His work friends were a big part of his social life. He felt a sense of belonging at work, and did not want to put any of it at risk with a relapse of depression.

I was in two minds about what to do next. Antidepressants are usually given to treat current depression, not future theoretical depression. And underlying this was the uncomfortable truth that SAD is a controversial diagnosis. It was first described in 1984 and, as its name suggests, is a cyclical disorder, occurring in the winter months when the days are short. Its symptoms are those of depression, although there are several differences. Firstly, there is (of course) a seasonal pattern. It starts to improve in spring and summer. And secondly, some of the features of SAD are not those of typical depression. Whereas depression is typically accompanied by insomnia, loss of appetite and weight loss, SAD is more commonly associated with hypersomnia (sleeping too much) and weight gain. These are symptoms of what is usually called 'atypical depression'.

The original 1984 study of SAD included twenty-nine patients, most of whom had an existing bipolar disorder.[13] The first patient, on whom the authors carried out a pilot study, was someone who had depression every winter and a kind of attenuated mania (called hypomania) every spring. Her cycles were affected by her latitude of residence, with depression worsening in more northerly latitudes (where it gets dark earlier, and is dark for longer, in autumn and winter). On two separate occasions, her winter depression disappeared within two days of a holiday in Jamaica. This led to the theory that the lack of sunlight was the cause of her winter depression. Other studies appeared to endorse the notion of SAD. A treatment for SAD based on light boxes was soon developed. These boxes look a bit like computer tablets, although they are designed to emit light of a certain intensity to replace the sunlight lacking in the winter months. Ron told me that he had already bought a light box, which he also hoped would reverse any effects of the shortening days. Yet he wanted the reassurance of having antidepressants on hand.

The problem is that there is a significant body of research that does not support the validity of SAD at all. One large US study of over 34,000 participants published in 2016 found no correlation of depression with either latitude, season or sunlight.[14] The authors concluded their paper with the comment, 'The idea of seasonal depression may be strongly rooted in folk psychology, but it is not supported by objective data.' This led to a reply from a researcher supportive of the diagnosis of SAD, who ended his piece with the rebuttal that the authors of the original study 'attempted to find a needle in a haystack with a faulty definition of the needle, a faulty definition of the haystack, and a faulty definition of "find"'.[15]

Yet since that exchange, further studies have been published again calling into question the validity of SAD as a separate entity. A Dutch study of over 5,000 people did not find much evidence for seasonal fluctuations in mood.[16] Researchers in Iceland, where there is a significant change in sunlight exposure between summer and winter, posted questionnaires in each of the four seasons to 1,000 randomly selected participants that asked them about their current mood.[17] Their concern was that many studies ask participants to remember their mood in the past, which has the potential for bias in favour of people remembering depression in winter. The researchers found no seasonal effect at all on either mood or anxiety. Careful not to go beyond the data, they concluded that for the Icelandic population at least, there is little propensity to seasonal mood changes, and no evidence for SAD.

A US study found that even mild depression was not associated with seasonal changes, latitude or daylight hours.[18] As for light boxes and light therapy, unfortunately the evidence is not convincing here either. *Cochrane Database of Systematic Reviews*, one of the most trusted resources for answering clinical questions, reviewed the published literature on light therapy.[19] The authors found no persuasive evidence that light therapy was effective, noting that the quality of evidence available was very low.

I think SAD has caused so much controversy because, intuitively, many people believe that there is a seasonal component to their mood. I am currently writing this chapter in the British Library in the middle of December, in an area with no natural light. On one side of me there is a whitewashed wall, and on the other side of me there is a wall of books behind a glass case, six floors high. The books are all ancient looking, dusty and with those orange-brown spines reminiscent of the library at Hogwarts, as if the right incantation will cause the correct book to dislodge itself from the shelves and fly through the air, landing with a thwack at my desk. The lighting is subdued. I entered the library a little after noon, and it is now 4 p.m. When I leave the library, which closes at 5 p.m. today, it will already be dark. This being a Sunday, and with work the next morning, I am feeling increasingly gloomy because the day feels like it's already over. There will be no barbeques or refreshing summer drinks on the lawn this evening, just the cold of a long winter's night, followed by a week at work.

Like many people, I start to feel more optimistic and energised in spring. I imagine if I were to answer a questionnaire next summer about my mood in winter, I would recall feeling gloomier at that time of the year. I would feel that life was somehow less colourful, more constrained, less enjoyable in winter. Whatever this feeling is, given that it is commonly experienced, could it be considered a diagnosis? To what extent should diagnoses be trying to capture some commonly felt, relatable human experience? This might fit into what Kendler refers to in his paper as 'coherence',[20] essentially that some diagnoses exist because they appear to fit with our observations about the world around us. As more information is gathered, perhaps correlation with brain imaging, neurochemical changes or genetic findings, the diagnosis can be refined. Yet I am not sure if this would work for a diagnosis of SAD, where the very premise of a seasonal component to mood is disputed. That approach may work better with something like bipolar disorder, where the observations of an individual's behaviour fit with existing scientific findings to form a coherent whole.

The percentage of the population said to have SAD is approximately 1–10%, depending on the latitude,[21] which is a huge number of people, and it again brings into question the boundary lines of depression and how we should think about SAD. Perhaps it is simply the way some humans react to diminished sunlight.

Certainly, the case for it being a form of depression is far from proven, yet in most cases that I have seen, people are prescribed antidepressants. In Ron's case, I decided in the end not to prescribe antidepressants. I could understand the rationale but I couldn't justify it to myself. I have doubts about the validity of the diagnosis and the wisdom of prophylactic antidepressant prescriptions. I imagine other doctors may have come to a different decision.

SAD is yet another factor adding to the demand for prescriptions of antidepressant medications, which in the UK has escalated significantly over recent years. In 2008, the number of prescriptions totalled 36 million. Only ten years later, in 2018, there were 70.9 million prescriptions and evidence of a steady, year-on-year increase in cases of depression.[22, 23] This figure does not include antidepressant prescriptions issued in private care, where – given the difficulties many patients have in accessing NHS care – millions more prescriptions would have been issued.

There is no doubt amongst clinicians who routinely treat depression that antidepressants do work, but the question is, who for? Well, the best place to look is the meta-analyses of antidepressants, which aggregate data from many different studies to draw even more robust conclusions. The conclusions are interesting but perhaps not surprising. Antidepressants are clearly effective, and the more severe the depression, the more effective they are.[24] Yet at mild levels of depression, their performance is often little better than a placebo. This leads us back to the discussion as to whether mild depression should be conceptualised differently. Whilst there needs to be some recognition that it is harder for an individual to function with even mild depression, thinking of it as an illness might not be justified, or helpful. It is a controversial argument to make, but in treating mild and severe depression in the same way, we dilute the argument for antidepressant treatment. And perhaps worse, it can mean that a person with more complex social and personal difficulties is given a pill because it's cheap and available.

I knew that I would do my best to treat Sian for her low mood, but deep down I wasn't very confident. Perhaps there would be some success, but I sensed that there were limits to how much any treatment would alter her perspective on life. Sometimes, the skill is knowing what is fixable and what isn't, and that is not always a clear line. If Sian kept coming back to doctor after doctor, it was surely more in hope than in expectation. But perhaps she herself wasn't expecting a cure. She was still here at least, and she still wanted help. Perhaps what she wanted most of all was to be able to talk to someone who understood. Is it an indictment of care if the patient needs more of it? Or should the need for long-term mental health care be seen like a diabetic's need for insulin, or a kidney patient's need for dialysis? People with physical health issues survive thanks to continuous treatment, and this is seen as medical success rather than failure.

One interesting study looked at the effect of therapists on recovery from depression independently of the type of therapy they were delivering. It showed that the personal qualities of the therapist themselves seemed to matter more than the type of therapy they were delivering.[25] There appeared to be something that good therapists were doing that transcended the formalities of the technique they were using. Experience and training seemed to count for relatively little, even though intuitively one might have expected them to matter more. Perhaps good therapists create a connection, inspire confidence or show an understanding and caring about the person sitting in front of them that the patient picks up on. It seems that few things are more therapeutic than being listened to and understood.

Treating depression can be hard to do well. It involves a curiosity and insight into people's lives – a deeper understanding of their symptoms and their meaning, their personalities, their coping and attributional styles, their support systems and their ability to respond constructively to crisis and adversity. Many cases of depression that I see would have been cases in any generation. Many, though, are far more nuanced and share a border with aspects of our normal daily experience. They sometimes reflect lives of disappointment, a lack of meaning and purpose, or thwarted ambition. I see other patients infused by a sense that they have been left behind and forgotten by the world, that in the scheme of things their lives don't matter. All of these are profoundly dispiriting things to consider.

In our time, in our culture, life is getting simultaneously better and worse. We have achieved a level of wealth and longevity that previous generations could only have dreamed about, and yet we have never been so unhappy. Depression is a diagnosis that has become emblematic of the early twenty-first century. Not a fashionable diagnosis, but a ubiquitous one.

The uneven rates of depression worldwide suggest we are picking up something beyond a biological illness. Life is beautiful and fragile, and all too brief. It is painful to think how many years are being lost to depression and unhappiness. Psychiatry holds only some of the answers. The rest needs to happen in a different way, assuming it matters enough to us. We need to be thinking about what in our culture is generating so much sadness. Framing this as depression is what is leading to the sharp rise in the diagnosis of depression and antidepressant prescription, and misses the point entirely.

7

Traumatised

Trauma has a strange history. In previous generations, the word 'trauma' was normally used to describe a physical injury.[1] If you told someone in the eighteenth century that you were traumatised, they would have had no idea what you meant, unless you were trying to tell them you had been shot or stabbed. Its use in a psychiatric setting only dates back to the late nineteenth century,[2] when the great French physician Jean-Martin Charcot developed the concept of psychic trauma.[3] Charcot had become famous for his studies on patients with hysteria.[4] At the time, although hysteria was well known, it was not considered a legitimate disease. It was commonly thought to be to do with women and their reproductive systems. Charcot, though, investigated it as a neurological illness. Patients presenting with symptoms of hysteria, such as strange fits and sudden weakness, were admitted to his hospital in Paris, the Salpêtrière. After analysing a series of patients with hysterical symptoms, Charcot posited that there must be a defect, a vulnerability within the individual. This would lie dormant until a triggering event, such as an assault or accident, which led to what he called 'traumatic hysteria'.[5] For the first time, trauma had gained traction as, at least in part, a mental and not just a physical injury.

Yet the term 'trauma' was slow to catch on in psychiatry. Even in as brutal a conflict as the First World War, the word trauma was not in common usage. 'Shell shock' came into being to describe the mental effects of war, initially thought to arise from a shell exploding near the unfortunate individual,[5] perhaps causing damage to the nerve cells. However, it became clear that soldiers nowhere near exploding ordnance had been affected too. Soon enough, shell shock came to be seen by the authorities as a sign of weakness, a character flaw or perhaps even cowardice in the face of the enemy. A 1922 British War Office report[6] cites an expert witness called to give evidence on shell shock. 'Frankly,' he states, 'I am not prepared to draw a distinction between cowardice and "shell shock" . . . "shell shock" to my mind [is] chronic and persisting fear.' The report goes on to recommend, 'The term shell-shock should be eliminated from official nomenclature.'

Everything changed in psychiatry in the 1970s, in the aftermath of the US's engagement in the Vietnam War. It was an unpopular, costly war that failed in its objectives, and anti-war protests were a staple of US culture in the late 1960s and early 1970s. Returning servicemen were greeted not as heroes but as instruments of an unjust conflict. Sympathy for their suffering was in short supply. Yet many of those servicemen began on their return to struggle with alcoholism, drugs, the breakdown of relationships and other long-term symptoms of distress.[7]

It was here that a new diagnosis was brought into being to account for their suffering – post-traumatic stress disorder, more commonly known as PTSD. This diagnosis had far more to do with political lobbying on behalf of the servicemen than any post-conflict research on psychiatric outcomes. Indeed, as Edgar Jones and Simon Wessely at King's College, London commented,[5] 'In part, validation of the disorder's [PTSD's] existence was a further way of undermining the US Government's pursuit of the war.' Undoubtedly, the other part was an attempt to gain some recognition for and legitimise the veterans' suffering.

The condition is now part of our collective understanding and its symptoms will be widely recognisable to the movie-going public. (The scene: the army locates a crack soldier at his remote farm. They need to persuade him to do one last vital mission. They fly the top brass out to make their case to him. The soldier is tending to his crops as he sees the whirring blades of the helicopter above him, and suddenly he's back in 'Nam. It's not just that he's remembering it, it's like he's actually there, re-experiencing all the chaos, fear and emotion that he experienced the first time around.)

People with PTSD are in a constant state of alert. They are hypervigilant and tense. They have vivid nightmares and, classically, immersive flashbacks of the traumatic event. These flashbacks are different from normal recollections; they have an emotional quality, a feeling of going through the event all over again.

And yet, within psychiatry, PTSD remains the subject of debate. A study[8] to address whether or not symptoms of PTSD have always existed but just remained unrecognised until the 1970s undertook a review of the service records of UK veterans of the Boer War, the First and Second World Wars and more recent conflicts. Records of individuals who had been awarded war pensions for post-combat disorders were selected randomly to see if any suffered from symptoms of PTSD. The authors of the study reasoned that if the condition has always existed, then key symptoms such as flashbacks would be evident in these records.

The researchers found that 'flashbacks were conspicuous by their absence in ex-servicemen from the Boer War and the First and Second World Wars'.[8] In other words, they found it unlikely that PTSD as a condition has always existed, at least in its current form. Symptoms of intrusion (a memory of an event that intrudes its way into your consciousness) and avoidance of reminders of the event, also staples of PTSD, again appear to be more modern representations of post-traumatic distress. This is not to say that war trauma did not exist – it undoubtedly had a substantial effect on the individuals exposed – but that its representation appears to have changed and its characteristics have been influenced by culture.

Regardless of the uncertainties around PTSD, it made its way into DSM-III in 1980, and the word 'trauma' entered the formal psychiatric lexicon for the first time.[3] In its original 1980s form, an incident considered sufficient to cause PTSD was something major and 'outside the range of normal human experience'.[9] PTSD was seen as arising from events that 'would evoke significant symptoms of distress in most people',[9] such as military combat, natural disasters, or severe assault.

Whether PTSD is useful as a diagnosis is very much a matter of perspective. It was certainly beneficial to some returning Vietnam veterans, whose psychological harm was formally recognised and validated. It was less helpful, though, to the large number of people who had been through all other kinds of misfortunes, both big and small, as it soon attracted legions of well-intentioned therapists who thought they could ameliorate or even prevent the disorder from developing. Soon, in the aftermath of any major incident, therapists would offer debriefing in an attempt to ward off PTSD. After the Concorde air crash in Paris, a team of counsellors were standing by. Similarly, after the shooting of Jean Charles de Menezes by police officers in a case of mistaken identity on the London Underground, counsellors were readied for action. The conceit is always the same – without therapists to guide us to emotional safety after an incident, we are all liable to fall into the abyss of PTSD.

It was, however, demonstrated that this kind of approach at best did nothing, and in some cases made people worse. A major review of the evidence for debriefing,[10] conducted by *Cochrane Database of Systematic Reviews*, concluded, 'There is no evidence that single session individual psychological debriefing is a useful treatment for the prevention of post traumatic stress disorder after traumatic incidents. Compulsory debriefing of victims of trauma should cease.' Yet, despite the evidence, the urge to debrief persisted. It was just too tempting a theory to give up, and made so much sense to the people delivering it that surely it had to be true. It was logical, easy to understand and allowed swift and decisive action after an unpleasant event. It would be like lancing a boil, releasing all that toxic emotion – those unpleasant memories and thoughts would be let out and everyday life could resume once more.

However, after a traumatic event, people will generally cope without the involvement of the caring professions. People will talk to friends or family,[11] or try to put it out of their minds. In other words, they will regain their mental equilibrium through their usual coping strategies. In some cultures, there is even the practice of 'active' or 'motivated' forgetting, a deliberate attempt to avoid any recollection of the event, as supported by a recent study that commented that 'forgetting is a hallmark of psychological well-being'.[12]

Active forgetting is at odds with our current culture, with the need to talk about problems rather than forget about them. But when it comes to traumatic events, it may help to think of traumatic memories as memories that won't behave like normal ones. With most memories, we can contextualise them, put them in the past, integrate them into the narrative of our lives. For traumatic events though, the memories cannot be integrated. They are endlessly relived in the present, with all the fear and emotions associated with the event. The problem with early debriefing after an unpleasant or traumatic event is that rehearsing the details whilst fresh in a person's mind can make them harder to forget. It is the exact opposite of what we are trying to achieve.

The other issue with debriefing is that it can undermine the individual by the implicit suggestion that they now have a problem needing professional help. It reinforces the idea that something potentially dangerous has happened to their psychological well-being that is no longer within their means to manage independently.

In spite of the ubiquity of the language of trauma, and the therapeutic industry that has grown up around it, there is still no real consensus on what psychological trauma might be. Whilst everyone understands, more or less, what physical trauma means, for psychological trauma, its original definition of an event out of the range of normal human experience has long since been abandoned by many of the people claiming expertise in the area.

So what is psychological trauma? Trauma, at its most elemental, could be conceived of as breaching a defence. This could be a physical defence, for example, in the case of a stabbing, where skin and bodily organs are breached. Or it could be a psychic defence, such as surviving a natural disaster like an earthquake, where the individual's ability to cope with the event has been exceeded. Yet it does not really have any formal definition, and this is where the problems have arisen.

I am in no doubt that there are some events that would count as deeply traumatic and cause symptoms that we would now call PTSD. However, since the psychological definition of trauma has always had unclear boundaries, what counts as traumatic has become entirely subjective. Increasingly, trauma is now what the person experiencing it perceives it to be. It has become a self-diagnosis, requiring only a declaration that one has been traumatised. After all, who is anyone to tell me what events in my life are traumatic? To give just one example, after an on-air row with her co-host Sharon Osbourne on US television, Sheryl Underwood believed she might have PTSD. In widely reported remarks, she said, 'I feel like I am in PTSD because it [the argument] was a trauma.'[13] Trauma has gone from the battlefield to the television studio, and from hostage-taking to hurt feelings.

It is hard to see how this change has been good for mental health. The word 'trauma' still has the power of the dangerous and threatening, and has not yet been diluted through overuse. It is well known that the words we use to describe something can significantly affect how we feel about that thing. In the 1970s, there was a famous study[14] in which students were asked to watch a video of a collision between two cars. They were then asked some questions about what they had seen. Some students were asked to estimate how fast the cars were going when they 'hit' one another. Others were asked to estimate how fast the cars were going when they 'collided', 'bumped into', 'made contact with' or 'smashed into' one another.

The study showed that if someone was asked how fast the cars were going when they 'smashed into' each other, they would estimate the speeds of the cars to be faster than those of the students asked the same question using 'hit', 'collided', 'bumped into' or 'made contact with'. There was another interesting conclusion to the study. One week later, the same students were asked if they recalled seeing any broken glass when they were shown the video of the collision. Those students who had been asked about the cars 'smashing into' each other were more likely to report seeing broken glass in the aftermath of the collision, even though there had been none in the video.

All of this shows how important our choice of words is in interpreting our experience. Using hyperbolic language to describe our past ('I was devastated, traumatised') may change what we remember and can colour our emotions and feelings towards those past experiences. Here, the caring professions can do much harm. When a patient comes to you with a life story of adversity and difficulty, the impulse may be to express empathy, but often the last thing they need to hear is that they were 'traumatised'. This official sanction and diagnosis can lead the unfortunate individual to see themselves as irreparably damaged. I see this in my clinics far too often, whereby a health professional has chosen to express their empathy in the language of trauma, adding to the patient's burden and perhaps even worsening their outcome. I have seen many diagnoses (schizophrenia, depression, anxiety) as well as distress attributed to trauma, and in most cases I do not think it adds any value to understanding the individual's suffering.

Gillian was a woman in her thirties who attended one of my outpatient clinics with a referral for depression. She was forthright and chatty as we walked from the waiting room, and this talkativeness continued into the consultation. It was hard for me to direct the narrative towards the subject that I wanted to ask about: the development of her depression. Eventually, the story of her life, until her messy divorce a year prior to the appointment, emerged. I began to think it could be seen in two different ways. One narrative would have been of a woman born to a working-class family, an only child, who was intelligent and ambitious and had decided against going to university and instead established a small business. She married and had two children, and she had by hard work and perseverance made a success of life.

Gillian's account of her life was very different. Her story was one of repeated setbacks, of being wronged, including by teachers at school, her friends and suppliers to her business. It was a narrative of struggle and grievance. That she had endured and overcome was seen by her not as personal growth in the face of life's challenges, but as a confirmation that we lived in a dog-eat-dog world. It had led to resentment and a jaundiced view of humankind.

It was after her husband told her that he had met someone else and wanted to end the marriage that her life started to fall apart. There was the house that needed to be sold and custody of the children to be resolved, and eventually the divorce turned into a contested and bad-tempered one, with blame and rancour all round. Throughout this process, her catering business had started to falter. Insolvency had happened, in a manner exactly like the famous Hemingway quote about bankruptcy, gradually and then suddenly.

As a backdrop to the development of depression, this seemed fertile ground, and it was understandable that she had been finding things a struggle. I tried to put together a treatment plan. As we talked about psychological and medication approaches, Gillian said she was already receiving therapy.

'Oh, that's good. What sort of therapy?'

'Trauma therapy.'

'Trauma therapy?' I wondered if I had missed something, a significant event that somehow hadn't come up in the consultation. Gillian stared at me for a moment, as though I hadn't been listening to a word.

'The divorce, the business, the whole thing.'

I nodded, but I wasn't quite sure I agreed. It seemed to me that Gillian's problem was not about reprocessing memories following a traumatic event, but about navigating the messy realities of her life. There was the change in circumstances, the loss of her business, her marriage, her financial security. It was also about her way of understanding the world, her sense of victimhood. To call the issues 'trauma' was to hide the complexity, to conceal rather than enlighten.

But trauma as a concept has become increasingly muddled. It is hard to know where the line is drawn now. There are the big-event traumas, such as wars and being taken hostage, and there are the day-to-day adversities like those Gillian had. Not trivial for her by any means, and clearly there were issues for her to work through. But to conceptualise them as trauma did, to my mind, deny an important aspect of Gillian's troubles. This was not about an event, the 'trauma', but rather about Gillian and her perception of her life and her coping strategies.

The idea of trauma is now commonly accepted and the language of trauma widespread. People are more likely to see themselves as traumatised by the more mundane and everyday adversities of life. And it works in reverse. Not only ordinary events but ordinary feelings are being attributed to 'trauma', so that if you work backwards from these feelings, it will lead you to the trauma that must have caused them.

The problem is that once an individual has come to see themselves as traumatised, it can be very difficult for a clinician in our current climate to disagree. It may be worth trying a thought experiment. Imagine you fell off a wall and broke your leg. You go to A&E, and the doctor confirms a traumatic fracture of your femur. Smiling brightly, they go on to tell you, 'It's good news though. It's not serious and you should recover before long.' You'd probably be pleased and quite relieved.

Now imagine that after falling off the wall you consider yourself psychologically troubled by the event. It was, after all, frightening and painful. You go to see the doctor, who listens to your story and then says, 'Yes, I can see that falling off the wall was distressing for you, and I understand you feel traumatised by it. But don't worry, it wasn't a serious trauma. You should be fine soon.' For some people, I imagine there would be a certain amount of surprise, possibly outrage. The doctor would be seen as not particularly sympathetic, not really listening, perhaps denying you the seriousness and reality of your feelings.

The language of trauma is a common currency on social media. Videos with titles such as 'Five signs you have trauma that you didn't know you had' can start to frame normal feelings and behaviours as the harbingers of mental illness. In a manner analogous to recovered memories, it can start to introduce the idea that the way you feel is because something has happened to you, something of which you were unaware. All of those unpleasant feelings you carried around with you are suddenly explained. The use of mental health terms in this way, to describe what usually has little to do with mental illness, has pernicious effects on the sense of well-being of vulnerable individuals watching. One video I was shown at a conference featured someone describing himself as a licensed therapist. He asked his audience, 'Are you hurting? If the answer is yes, you have trauma, and don't let anyone tell you that you're not.' It's hard to know where to start with this. What does 'hurting' even mean? And what does 'trauma' mean? And why not let someone tell you that you don't have trauma, if they have the appropriate expertise? Such videos might look plausible and seem compassionate if you take them at face value. Yet they are the inverse of compassion. And by watching to the end of the video, the algorithms ensure that wobbling individuals are served up with more of the same.

There are few more representative examples of the current concern for trauma than 'trigger warnings'. Most of us will now be familiar with trigger or content warnings, which alert listeners or viewers that the content they are about to engage with may re-activate or exacerbate mental health problems. Undoubtedly, they were introduced out of kindness and consideration, very much in keeping with our current cultural climate. Yet, a recent study suggests the opposite, that trigger and content warnings increase anxiety in anticipation of the warned-about event and make no difference to the emotional response to it.[15]

A separate study[16] explored the responses to trigger warnings of those considered trauma survivors or participants with a probable

PTSD diagnosis. Again, it found no evidence that trigger warnings were helpful. Perhaps worse though, trigger warnings were thought to be countertherapeutic since they 'reinforce[d] survivors' view of their trauma as central to their identity'.[16] Yet it seems that evidence has taken second place to what has become a compassionate-sounding cultural habit, developed with the best of intentions, that provides either no benefit or actually causes harm.

The cases where trauma has been unmistakable are often the ones I think about years later. Stories of torture, war or accidents in which the person believes that they are unlikely to survive – these are the infrequent but haunting accounts I hear from patients that can lead to PTSD. I remember seeing Martin, a man in his thirties who had been speeding on the motorway. He was unable to brake in time when he realised that the traffic ahead had slowed. He swerved to avoid the car in front and hit a barrier, and his car overturned. He told me that his upturned car skidded along the motorway for some time, with a metallic shuddering and scraping as the roof dragged along the tarmac. He couldn't see anything and had lost his bearings entirely. As his car eventually began to slow, he realised he was stuck inside it. He could hear the noise of other cars passing at motorway speeds, and was certain that it was only a matter of moments before one smashed into him and ended his life. In that moment he experienced a profound and existential fear of his imminent death. It was this fear that he could no longer rid himself of, long after he had been safely rescued.

He felt frightened leaving his flat, in case he heard sounds that reminded him of his car skidding on its roof. These included the nearby train tracks, where the screech of trains filled him with dread. He felt constantly on alert, vigilant for any threats around him. He began to worry about people breaking into his flat, being followed, and his safety out on the street.

He told me he had recently become single. His girlfriend could no longer tolerate his moods. There was an irritability and argumentativeness that were not part of the person she knew. And neither had he previously been a timid or anxious person. He just couldn't seem to break free of this persistent fear that hung over him in the day and followed him into his dreams at night.

Even though he had come to see me, he was reluctant to get the help that he needed. Medication can play a role in managing PTSD, but that was not an avenue he wanted to explore. Some patients just don't like the idea of psychotropic medication, and I can sympathise with this. In my experience, beyond explaining the rationale for prescription and the potential benefits and drawbacks, little good comes of trying to force the issue. We discussed the role of psychological therapies in managing PTSD, in processing the memories and emotions around the event and in helping with the avoidance and withdrawal that symptoms can cause. Yet Martin had a reluctance to engage in therapy that he was never fully able to explain. He said that he just didn't believe in it. I suggested a different form of therapy, known as eye movement desensitisation and reprocessing (EMDR), that would not involve him having to talk about the event that day on the motorway, but he didn't want that either. We were left in the position of him coming to see me every few weeks, but without any active treatment taking place between appointments. He wanted reassurance that he wasn't 'going mad' and that he would eventually get better. Over the six months that I saw him, I wasn't really sure he had. Sometimes PTSD gets better without treatment and sometimes it doesn't. In the end, I discharged him from the clinic and left the door open for him to come back and see me if he did want treatment.

Some months later he did come back, this time after his family had insisted that he needed help. After some discussion, he started EMDR, a therapy now thirty years old but which remains somewhat mysterious in its mechanism of action, despite the number of theories about why it works.[17] It involves making side-to-side eye movements whilst focusing the mind on the traumatic event. In some way, this seems to diminish the emotions associated with it and help reprocess the traumatic memory. Martin also wanted to try some medication, which I ended up giving alongside the EMDR. Over the following months, his symptoms steadily began to ease, and his life finally started to return to normal. By the time I discharged him for the second time, he was able to go out of the house without fear and have a social life again.

Psychological trauma can have significant consequences for individuals exposed to extreme events, and the road back can be long and painful, as it was for Martin. People can develop serious psychological impacts in response to shocking and life-threatening events. Yet in the public discourse, there has been a muddling of terms, an increasing looseness to the word 'trauma', with the language of diagnosis used without conveying any diagnostic meaning, which tends to hide rather than enlighten. When this term is used more loosely and becomes the focus, the difficult work of understanding why the person has reacted in a certain way can get lost. There is an increasing use of the word to describe events, which comes from social media, and often from therapists and doctors, and it is the language of sympathy and kindness, but I am far from convinced that it is helpful. And it is hard to see how we will reconcile the diagnostic classifications with the lay use of 'trauma' any time soon.

I wonder how historians of medicine will look back on this time, with trauma as an explanatory model capturing all in its embrace. Perhaps physicians in times gone by also realised the shortcomings of the four-humours theory, and deep down had their doubts about the benefits of leeches, cupping and purges. Perhaps my eighteenth-century colleagues rolled their eyes when the latest pamphlet made the case for animal magnetism, and hoped that physicians in the future would be a little more discerning. So, to my physician readers in the future, like you, we are navigating our own messy cultural context and trying to find our way forward.

8

The Rise (and Rise) of
Neurodevelopmental Disorders

I spend too much time on X/Twitter. It's a way of idling my brain in neutral in an attempt to ease the cares of life. Except that it never works like that. The debates are poorly informed, polarised and designed to keep a certain level of outrage bubbling away. I write measured and dignified replies to some of the more outlandish comments and then delete them, because what's the point? It reminds me of a cartoon I saw once, where there's a man sitting in his study on his computer. Someone in the background is imploring him to come to bed. 'I can't,' he says, 'someone is wrong on the internet.'[1]

Even if the debates shed more heat than light, what X/Twitter is good at is telling you something about where we are culturally. We have all been encouraged to take sides in the culture wars, and the posts presented to us often confirm our own biases. It is the worst sort of way to understand the world, with an inherent bias built into the arguments we see, so that too often our starting point for a topic is our own conclusions, before we have really heard the other side.

It was in this context that a cartoon credited to Doug Bratton appeared in my own feed. It depicted the beds of the seven dwarves from *Snow White*. Each of the dwarves had their name at the foot of the bed, only each name had been crossed out and replaced. Where Happy slept, the sign now read 'Euphoric'. Grumpy's name had been replaced with 'Depressed', 'Sleepy' had become 'Narcoleptic', 'Sneezy' was now 'Allergic', 'Dopey' was 'Mentally Challenged', and 'Bashful' had become 'Social Anxiety Affected'.[2] It was perhaps unfair, but it did seem to reflect something of a wider truth. Those character traits that we had previously acknowledged as common and part of life's rich tapestry have now become pathologised and medicalised. Not only that, but the diagnostic labels are starting to become part of people's public – or at least online – identity.

I suspect this phenomenon can be traced back in part to what is commonly referred to as identity politics, in which individuals of marginalised groups find belonging and meaning in an identity. With the breakdown of the previous social and religious structures that gave people a sense of their place in the world, identity is sought in other ways. Generally, these identities have been based on ethnicity, culture, race, sexuality. But more and more, they are based on medical diagnoses too. I have commonly seen X/Twitter profiles, which are limited to a few staccato words or phrases, that include someone's mental health diagnosis. Rather than it being a private matter, people are taking public ownership of it. In many ways, this is laudable and is indicative of how far we have come from the days of stigma. But this quintessentially modern approach to mental health and mental illness also seems strangely regressive. Why would anyone want a diagnostic label to be the first thing someone sees or knows about them? Surely people are all more nuanced and complex than to be contained or summed up in a single diagnostic label. Haven't anti-stigma campaigners spent decades fighting for the idea that individuals are more than just a label?

It is interesting that certain diagnoses are more readily worn as identities than others. I can imagine an X/Twitter biography that says, 'Teacher; mother of three girls; Wigan Athletic; ADHD'. I cannot imagine it saying, 'Nurse; West Ham; schizophrenia' or 'Taxi driver; father of two; persecutory delusions'.

It is not clear how some diagnoses infiltrate the public consciousness, but it seems that in psychiatry, as well as in general medicine, certain criteria need to be met. The first is that the diagnostic criteria need to be broad, flexible and subjective. This means that the severity or even the presence of symptoms is measured by what the person experiencing them says, rather than any agreed and laid-down criteria. The second is that the diagnostic criteria overlap with many aspects of normal human experience, and so what is being discussed is a difference in degree, rather than a difference in kind. And finally, gaining the diagnosis needs to have an explanatory function, in this case helping people make sense of their lives through the lens of the diagnosis.

Attention deficit hyperactivity disorder (ADHD) in adults is one such diagnosis. I would estimate that of every ten patients that I see in my clinics, approximately two or three have wondered about, or been advised by friends or family to ask about, adult ADHD as an explanation for their troubles. It may happen when I am treating someone for depression, or an anxiety disorder, or issues tangentially related to sleep, or really any psychiatric assessment. Sometimes the suggestion is made at the outset of the consultation, although more commonly it is a question that arises as I am summing up. I can often see why the patient may have wondered about ADHD as a diagnosis, although it's far less often that I find myself agreeing with it. Whenever it is mentioned, ADHD tends to upend the consultation. Whilst I am trying to distil the patient's complaints and experiences into a diagnostic formulation that accounts for the symptoms, their personality, the context of their lives, ADHD comes along like a wrecking ball, levelling the field again. The diagnosis must be considered fairly, a time-consuming process in itself, and in those circumstances where a case could be made for it, it is often in the context of other personality factors or psychiatric diagnoses that would make a new diagnosis of ADHD unwise, since treatment of the other diagnoses may make the ADHD-type symptoms melt away.

Adult ADHD was a diagnosis that barely existed a generation ago. During my training, ADHD was largely a diagnosis made in children. The first time I heard about it being applied to adults was in 2000, at a lunchtime neuropsychiatry meeting. One of the senior clinicians had developed an interest in it. He explained, to a somewhat sceptical audience, what the diagnosis was and how it was made, and speculated that it was under-diagnosed. The 'awareness raising' of the diagnosis was obviously happening elsewhere too, although at the time it seemed a rather niche area, a rare oddity in the psychiatric lexicon.

We were all familiar with childhood ADHD, of course. This was one of the disorders grouped under the label of 'neurodevelopmental disorders'. Which is to say, they are disorders that become apparent as the brain develops, when the behavioural and cognitive deficits are gradually exposed by abnormal brain development. They are therefore usually diagnosed in childhood, and the symptoms are not difficult to notice. They are broadly divided into two categories: inattentiveness, or lack of focus; and hyperactivity including impulsiveness. In the first category of inattentiveness, children are careless, make mistakes all the time, don't concentrate in class at school and are disorganised, with little perseverance for tasks that require more discipline and focus. The second category, the hyperactivity aspect, is even more obvious, with constant fidgetiness and restlessness and, at school, children unable to restrain themselves from cutting across conversations to say their piece without waiting for their turn to talk, interrupting the whole time and, in the same vein, acting without thinking.

This will get children into scrapes, particularly because of a lack of regard for personal danger. A child with ADHD could likely be correctly identified by any teacher in a class – and probably by the other children too.

There is good evidence though that some of the ADHD symptoms seen in childhood are not necessarily caused by a brain with a neurodevelopmental issue. They could be a sign of immaturity. One study showed that for children with August birthdays, who were the youngest in the class (where the school year begins in September), there was a significant increase in the rate of ADHD diagnosis.[3] The difference a year makes in a child's development can be substantial. And in some cases, these differences in maturity levels were wrongly attributed to ADHD, which is a worry, given that a prescription for stimulant medication such as amphetamines often follows.

There has always been a question about whether ADHD persists into adulthood or if it is essentially a disorder of childhood, with the neurodevelopmental issues generally resolving over time as the brain develops. One highly cited paper set out to answer this by exploring the drop-off in rates of ADHD diagnosed in childhood. It was a meta-analysis, the type of study that amalgamates lots of other published studies to make the results more powerful. What it showed was that if by 'persisting into adulthood' we meant meeting the full diagnostic criteria for ADHD in adulthood, then only 15% of cases diagnosed in childhood persisted into adulthood, supporting the notion that, at least in its full form, it is primarily a condition of childhood.[4]

The authors allowed for the fact that perhaps the sensitivity of adult criteria was not sufficient to pick up adult ADHD, and also acknowledged that many of the cases of adult ADHD had partially rather than fully resolved symptoms. Yet the study went some way to confirm what we already knew, which is that whilst many children grow out of it, some cases of childhood ADHD persist into adulthood. A minority of these are in the full form, with other cases persisting in a watered-down way. But what about ADHD that seems to arise for the first time in adulthood? This is proving to be one of the fastest-growing areas in psychiatry and is a cause for concern. The NHS has simply buckled under the tsunami of ADHD referrals. A recent news report revealed that in many areas of the UK, the waiting list for assessment was at least eight years, with at least 196,000 adults now waiting for an assessment in the UK.[5]

A BBC documentary interviewed a GP, who spoke of the day-to-day, practical problem of so many people believing they may have ADHD. When asked about the scale of it, she replied that the number of people seeking an assessment of ADHD was 'of the order of at least twenty times more people coming now than there were five or six years ago'.[6] I think every doctor in the country watching would have been nodding along in agreement, because when I speak to my colleagues about it, we all recount very similar experiences. In a recent post on a forum for UK doctors, a GP said that in around 40% of their consults that day, the person attending the appointment wanted to know if their problems (ranging from insomnia to anxiety to hot flushes) were attributable to ADHD. Many other doctors added that their experiences were similar.

With NHS capacity overwhelmed, there has been a mushrooming of private clinics specialising in ADHD. The BBC documentary was an investigative report to see whether there was any truth in the perception, advanced by desperate patients attending these clinics, of the low quality of some of the assessments being offered by private clinics. The reporter began the documentary by attending a full three-hour assessment from an expert psychiatrist working in a specialist ADHD service in the NHS.

After what sounded like an exhausting appointment, the journalist was told that he did not have ADHD, despite a number of suggestive symptoms. Three separate video assessments from private clinics all concluded that he did.

What the fuller assessment did was to contextualise his symptoms and understand them in the context of his underlying personality, life story and other relevant factors. The assessments that confirmed ADHD, by contrast, seemed to offer a tick-box approach to diagnosis, where symptoms were seen as isolated entities with no context. My own experience of seeing patients who have come to me from private clinics is that in nearly all cases, if they have gone to a private clinic to investigate a potential ADHD diagnosis, they have had an ADHD diagnosis endorsed.

One study, published in the *American Journal of Psychiatry*, examined the rates of ADHD in a group born in New Zealand in 1972–73, who were followed up until they were age thirty-eight.[7] Firstly, they looked at those people diagnosed in childhood to see what had happened to them. They found that, like in the study above, there was a small persistence of ADHD into adulthood (6%), which was lower than that in the earlier study and predominantly in men. But what was really interesting and novel was that the study also examined the issue from the other way around. The researchers looked at individuals diagnosed for the first time in adulthood, finding a rate of ADHD diagnosed in adulthood of 3%, this time with an equal gender balance. They then went back to the earlier records to see whether there was any evidence of it in childhood. They found that the adult-diagnosed group did not have the same characteristics as the childhood group, and that 90% of the diagnosed adults did not have a history of childhood ADHD. The researchers stated in their summary of results, 'Unexpectedly, the childhood ADHD and adult ADHD groups comprised virtually nonoverlapping sets.'

'Unexpected' is about as strong an adjective as an academic paper permits itself. It really was a striking finding and raises the question, what is adult ADHD? How can it be the same neurodevelopmental disorder as childhood ADHD if most of those diagnosed have no neurodevelopmental problems? In fact, how can it be a neurodevelopmental disorder at all? And if not neurodevelopmental, then what is adult ADHD? What is this phenomenon that we are now seeing? To answer these questions, it is worth considering how the diagnosis is commonly made.

Like all psychiatric diagnoses, the diagnosis of ADHD is first of all considered in light of the symptoms that the patient reports. The NHS website on ADHD is very good and sets out a symptom checklist.[8] Symptoms include the usual ones of impulsivity, disorganisation and inattentiveness that characterise the diagnosis. The website also warns that symptoms in adults can be far more subtle than those in children, which means the symptoms associated with adult ADHD can be subtle, common and relatable to the daily lives of most people. One academic paper, commenting on the diagnostic criteria for ADHD, stated, 'The DSM-5 criteria for adult ADHD are so broad that they fail to distinguish between illness and normal variation.'[9] If the practitioner is hasty or inexperienced, or relies solely on the number of ticks against the checklist, it is easy to see why many people are meeting the criteria for a diagnosis. It has to be acknowledged too that the burgeoning private sector market for ADHD assessments seems to be focused as much on income as on good medical care, and this can mean keeping attendees satisfied by giving them the diagnosis they think they want.

I saw Gary in an afternoon clinic. He was forty, the referral said, with a failed marriage behind him, and now living with his girlfriend of two years in a somewhat tempestuous relationship. He had been referred with depression and suicidal thoughts, and his unease at being at the appointment was apparent as soon as we met. I was also struck by the fact that he kept apologising, starting with when I let him into the room ahead of me, then after he put his cup of water on the desk between us, and after putting his bag on the chair next to him. He then apologised because he hardly knew where to start in telling me of his problems, so we went back to the beginning.

His father had been a peripheral presence in his childhood, sparing with praise and seemingly without paternal feelings towards Gary, who tried everything he could to please him, but it was never enough. His mother was herself depressed, and used alcohol to manage her emotions. When Gary's father left, she became caught up in the dramas of her own life, and soon prioritised her drinking over her children. Gary had few happy memories of his childhood, didn't much care for school and was pleased when he finally left home. He had a brother and a sister, both younger, with whom he was close.

He told me that over the years he'd had recurrent depression, and on one occasion in his early twenties had taken an impulsive overdose when life had been getting on top of him. He had always regretted doing that. He thought in retrospect that he had been depressed at the time, but his depression hadn't yet been diagnosed, and he had feared that this was how his life was going to be, and he said he couldn't take it. But he was soon treated and he put the episode behind him.

Life ticked along. He had always worked in traffic management. He married in his mid-twenties, but his recurrent depression seemed to weigh heavily on the relationship, which eventually faltered and then came to an end after a brief admission to hospital for treatment of his depression. He had a son from the marriage whom he saw from time to time, but not as often as he would have liked.

He was now depressed again, with typical depressive symptoms. He was miserable, unable to work and didn't want to see any of his friends. He admitted to feeling trapped and helpless in his situation, unable to see himself ever getting better. He had frequent thoughts that it would be better if he just went to sleep and didn't wake up in the morning. His self-esteem was at rock bottom ('I'm a waste of space') and he lacked energy and motivation. His libido had evaporated. ('We haven't done it in months,' he told me, although added that he wasn't much bothered.)

We agreed his depression needed properly treating, and I started by changing his antidepressants. I had expected a slow and gradual improvement, so it was a surprise to see him much better at his next appointment around a month later. But, like all dramatic recoveries in psychiatry, in my experience at least, they can often be quite brittle. True to form, the next time I saw Gary he was much worse again, triggered by an argument with his girlfriend. He told me a neighbour had called the police because of the noise, and he felt deeply ashamed. His mood fluctuated over the next few months, before eventually stabilising, with life starting to return to normal.

When we next met, he wanted to discuss something else. His girlfriend had told him she thought he might have ADHD, and so he wanted to know if I could check him out for that. At the appointment, he told me about a number of ADHD-like symptoms that had been there since childhood. He was a daydreamer at school, found it hard to focus on lessons and was careless with details of classwork and homework. He was fidgety and found it hard to sit still, a trait that continued into adulthood. As an adult, he would sometimes find himself cutting across conversations when he thought of something to say, without waiting his turn to speak. At work, he found it difficult to do tasks that required sustained attention, or complete jobs that he started before moving to the next one.

On the face of it, he did seem to have symptoms of ADHD. Yet his symptoms seemed to be conflated with his depression and anxiety, as well as those personality and coping styles he had developed in a childhood of rejection and adversity. I also noted that these symptoms are common in the population. Avoiding difficult tasks in favour of easier ones, or cutting across someone to talk, or not engaging at school may also be signs of normality. We discussed what to do next, and he decided to seek an ADHD assessment. He returned some months later with a thoughtful report, which eventually concluded, notwithstanding the reservations about his other diagnoses, that ADHD was present, and stimulant medication, the standard treatment for ADHD, was prescribed.

He took the stimulants for months, but they made almost no difference to his symptoms. I wasn't particularly surprised. He then began to wonder if ADHD really was the diagnosis, or whether his symptoms could be better explained by a different diagnosis. I understood his need to make sense of his life and his need for a diagnosis that explained why he thought and behaved the way he did. Yet I had my reservations about the direction his treatment was taking. He ended up having an online consultation with a doctor from the US whom he had found in an internet search, and the last time I saw him, he was considering going to a retreat there.

Gary is typical of a number of my patients now, who have come to wonder whether there is a unifying diagnosis that can contain and explain all that doesn't feel right about their life. Thanks to the breadth of its criteria, and the fact that they overlap with so many areas that are for many people a common experience, it is easy to see how ADHD can fit the bill.

At a population level, there is no doubt that diagnoses of ADHD have been rising sharply, both in adults and in children. To appreciate the scale of the problem, it may be worth starting with the rate of diagnosis of ADHD in children. The US Centers for Disease Control and Prevention (CDC) has graphics showing the rate of diagnosis of ADHD, using the National Health Interview Survey data from 1997 to 2018.[10] The rate in children is about 5–6% in 1997, and climbs steadily over time to about 10% in 2018. This is a very large increase, particularly when thinking about how many children this represents. Notably, the survey includes children as young as three years old, far younger than ever used to be thought capable of displaying ADHD symptoms. Some of the increased rate of diagnosis is likely to be due to better awareness and targeting the right children. My sense though is that, like for the August birthdays, there is a large cohort of children in there whose diagnosis is far less robust and who really don't belong.

As to adults, ADHD was rarely diagnosed in adults a generation ago, and something not even considered except as a continuation of childhood illness. In fact, the diagnostic criteria specify that the forerunners of the adult illness need to have been present in childhood. Yet we have seen that this is not true for most adults diagnosed with ADHD. A study in the US in 2006 put the rate of adult ADHD at 4.4% of the population.[11]

Increased rates of ADHD diagnosis and prescription are not by definition a bad thing. It just depends on who is being diagnosed and on what grounds. I have seen in my own clinics people whose lives have been transformed by a competently made diagnosis of ADHD followed by effective treatment, which can bring stability to their lives, improve their ability to sustain employment and allow them to become more productive. Yet the difficulty of diagnosing adult ADHD is that it exists on a spectrum from behaviour that is essentially a variant of normal to something that is clearly beyond the usual norms. And because symptoms are so diffuse, they can easily overlap with other mental health diagnoses such as anxiety disorders, bipolar disorder, OCD or personality disorders. When a symptom-checklist approach to diagnosing ADHD is used, the other disorders are likely to be missed and an erroneous diagnosis of ADHD made instead.

Another aspect of the problem is that narratives in psychiatry tend to be about under-diagnosis rather than over-diagnosis. 'Awareness raising' campaigns usually involve campaigners for their particular diagnosis exhorting the medical profession not to miss diagnoses and so fail patients. Many GPs have a slight dread of such campaigns, as they anticipate their surgeries becoming full of people identifying with the symptoms, and they will come under pressure to agree with the diagnosis and either prescribe medication or refer them to specialist clinics.

One of the arguments put forward for adult diagnoses of ADHD is that of 'masked symptoms'. This is a relatively new concept. The theory is that some people, particularly girls, are more able to conceal or suppress their symptoms by copying social norms and observing what others are doing, accounting for why they are more likely to present for the first time in adulthood. One expert in ADHD I spoke to was sceptical of the notion. 'What does it [masking] mean? How can you mask hyperactivity?' The ability to suppress our behaviours is often required to be part of normal society, and the successful ability to mask our thoughts, impulses, behaviours and actions is how we learn to become social beings and get along in the world.

The same specialist spoke of his unease about not giving someone the diagnosis that they have expected to receive, particularly when they have waited for years to be seen. Individuals may have started to construct their lives around the narrative of an ADHD diagnosis, and many will have joined support groups to become part of a community of fellow sufferers. He told me that during a consultation, as the patient's history unfolds and he becomes increasingly confident that ADHD is not the diagnosis, an anxiety begins to take hold of how he is going to break it to the patient. Those denied the diagnosis are often unhappy not to have been given it – a strange inversion of the normal run of events – and may feel that they are not being heard, or that their symptoms are not being taken seriously. There is a clash between what the patient wants and what the doctor believes. In an increasingly consumer-driven healthcare system, this can cause problems. Those with the ability to do so may seek another opinion. But in the moment, it can lead to a difficult and unsatisfactory consultation.

Lost in the discussion is the fact that, when making a diagnosis like ADHD, what matters more than the symptoms is their effects. We have become unable to see the wood for the trees. When an individual is managing in their professional life and home life, meaning their symptoms are not in any meaningful way holding them back, then one has to question whether their symptoms really qualify as a disorder. In other words, for someone who has symptoms – or behaviour traits – that are mild, whose life is not significantly impaired, this leads to a diagnostic conundrum, a grey area where societal values start to take precedence over diagnostic boundaries. If the prevailing view is that no symptoms should be allowable, if any deviation from the expected is sufficient to qualify for a diagnosis or warrant treatment, then we can soon find ourselves in a situation where increasingly few people would qualify for normal health. This is a problem highlighted by the former head of the DSM task force Allen Frances in his book *Saving Normal*,[12] referring to the 'huge epidemics of ADHD, autism, and bipolar disorder'.

Frances argues that part of the blame for the sharp rise in the number of ADHD diagnoses lies with pharmaceutical companies looking to expand their market into ADHD with their newly patented medications. In the US, it is common to see television advertisements sponsored by pharmaceutical companies badgering viewers to 'ask your physician to prescribe [our new and patented wonderdrug]'. This direct-to-consumer advertising undoubtedly makes a difference to prescribing habits, as the pressure comes now from the patient, and sometimes for busy clinicians, the path of least resistance is the easiest one to travel.

In the UK, we are somewhat shielded from the excesses of pharmaceutical advertising. There is no direct advertising to patients, and in many hospital trusts, there is a somewhat puritanical refusal to have drug-company-sponsored lunches. The pharmacy-sponsored inducements for the average doctor were never that appealing in the first place. I remember clearly when, on the same day that an old school friend of mine got a bonus from his bank of almost £200,000, after six years of medical school and two years as a doctor, I got a slinky, one of those helical springs that you can make walk downstairs (if you get the distance from the edge of the top step to the next step down just right) with the drug name printed on the side of the box. Usually though, it was a cheap plastic pen, or some Post-it notes. Soon it was nothing at all, aside from a Marks & Spencer cheese sandwich to sustain you for the academic meeting, until drug-sponsored lunches were banned completely, and we were back to eating curly egg-and-cress sandwiches from hospital catering, with that weird sort of tangy mayonnaise they always had, and the sides of the bread dry from being left out all morning.

It would be naive though to think that the pharmaceutical industry hasn't profited in the UK, or played its own role in advancing diagnoses for which it has patented treatments. Because the sales tactics are less high-pressured, we tend to be exposed less to the other behind-the-scenes goings-on that lead to higher drug sales. These have included the use of opinion leaders to persuade the profession of the need for increased diagnosis and prescription, and the ghostwriting of academic papers. There have also been reports of grassroots patient groups being funded by drug companies to lobby the National Institute for Health and Care Excellence to approve their drugs.[13] Whether or not there has been any industry involvement with ADHD, it is a fact that the sharp rise in drug prescriptions for ADHD has matched the sharp rise in diagnosis. A UK study showed that the prevalence of ADHD drug use in children increased thirty-four-fold from 1995 to 2008 before stabilising.[14] A study from Ireland, looking at prescribing rates even over the relatively recent past, showed that the number of children being prescribed ADHD medication had more than doubled from 2005 to 2015.[15] Prescription rates for ADHD vary worldwide, with rates of prescriptions of stimulant medication for children of 0.27% in France in 2010 and 6.69% in the US, and those in adults varying from 0.003% in Japan to 1.48% in the US.[16] These figures are surely saying something about the cultural as well as the medical aspects of managing symptoms.

Sometimes, the fact that the drugs work for ADHD is taken as a retrospective endorsement of the diagnosis. Although this intuitively makes sense, it is not necessarily true. Stimulants (the medications used in ADHD) can make many people feel better – sharper and more alert. When an adult who has received a diagnosis of ADHD feels better on the medication, it is hard to tell whether it is the medication treating an underlying condition, or whether it is just the general effects of the treatment, which would give anyone a lift. On that point, there have been concerns expressed of healthy individuals feigning or exaggerating symptoms of ADHD so that they can get a prescription of stimulants. This may be for a variety of reasons including weight loss, improved athletic performance or academic accommodation (such as being allocated extra time in exams), as well as the potential benefit for exam performance.[17]

In addition, if the diagnostic boundaries become ever wider, the diagnosis will cease to carry the same meaning. It will attract scepticism from otherwise supportive people, and an assumption that ADHD is not quite a real diagnosis. And of course, there is the question of what this will mean for research. If new treatments or diagnostic tools are being tested in such a heterogeneous population, where mild cases are lumped in with severe ones under the same ADHD label, will it dilute the conclusions reached from whatever is being studied, be it the underlying genetics, the diagnostic criteria or new treatments?

ADHD is not the only neurodevelopmental diagnosis that has become increasingly visible. Thanks in part to a change in the diagnostic boundaries, many patients find themselves wondering about autism. Linda was a middle-aged woman who had worked for at least twenty years in an estate agency, taking prospective buyers to see new properties and trying to complete sales or rental agreements. She was married and had a grown-up son, whom she was close to. Over the years, she had been intermittently prone to anxiety, which was sometimes treated by her GP with a course of anti-anxiety medication, and sometimes it would seem to clear up on its own. This time though, and without particular reason, her anxiety had taken a hold and not let go. During the consultation, we tried to make sense of this seemingly capricious illness. We explored possible triggers, the stresses in her life, all the interpersonal and other events that make up a life, that might induce prolonged anxiety. Really though, there wasn't too much to go on. It sometimes happens like this. There is a biological reality to some illnesses that they don't seem to have a cause other than that they just are. We always go looking to understand why something has happened now, at this time and in this way, yet sometimes we have to accept that illness and emotions don't always run along a logical narrative.

Treatment, though, had been progressing reasonably well. There had already been some improvement in Linda's anxiety, albeit still with a little way to go. The mainstay of her treatment had been finding an effective medication and titrating the dose to the right level. In some ways, it was what psychiatrists might think of as a bread-and-butter case. But after three or four appointments, Linda asked if her symptoms could be caused by undiagnosed autism. 'I get anxious when I talk to other people,' she told me. 'I think they don't really like me. I never know what to say.' She told me she didn't always read other people well, that she didn't have many friends. People had commented that she could be quite direct in her speech. She explained that busy or crowded social situations made her feel quickly overwhelmed.

Given that the concept of autism is changing, it is understandable that patients pick up on the changes and wonder if it applies to them. There is more about the diagnosis on social media and in the press, and an increasing number of people seem to be diagnosed with it. A large study in the US by the CDC showed that in under fifteen years, the rate of diagnosis in children over the age of eight had more than doubled from one in 150 children in 2000–2002 to one in sixty-eight in 2010–2012, increasing yet further to one in fifty-nine by 2014.[18] Another study based in the US, this time looking at ASD in children and adolescents aged three to seventeen, found prevalence rates of 2.79% (one in thirty-six) in 2019 and 3.49% (one in twenty-nine) in 2020.[19]

Children who would now be described as autistic have always been with us, although initially they were thought of, in the early part of the twentieth century, as having a form of childhood schizophrenia.[20] It was not until 1980, as the understanding of it advanced, that a separate category of autism made it into the diagnostic classification DSM-III.[21] The diagnosis of autism included significant intellectual or learning difficulties, and this is how it was (and is) commonly thought of. Occasionally one would come across people known as 'savants', made famous by Dustin Hoffman's portrayal of Raymond Babbitt in the film *Rain Man*. Whilst savants have the usual difficulties common to all autism, there is an area of outstanding intellectual ability, nearly always involving memory, such as (in the case of Raymond Babbitt) memorising a telephone book, or card counting (when in the casino – the dramatic centre of the film). The reality for most people with autism, though, is of a disorder that is apparent by the age of three, with significant developmental delay, extreme difficulties understanding social interaction, problems with communication and what is described in the ICD classification as 'restricted, stereotyped, repetitive behaviour'. Other behavioural disturbances are commonly seen, including temper tantrums and aggression (typically directed towards themselves).

For many years, there was another category in the diagnostic classifications, which was seen as related but separate from autism, called Asperger's syndrome. I think many of us would recognise the description from someone we know or have met. People with this syndrome are of normal intelligence but might prefer solitary pastimes and find social interactions challenging. They can be literal, not understanding nuance or reading between the lines of a conversation. They can struggle to read facial expressions. People with Asperger's syndrome would not, for example, easily be able to tell if they are boring the other person or causing offence, or whether they had misjudged a situation entirely and said the wrong thing. These difficulties in reading social interactions can be a real challenge in life – all the workplace meetings, office politics and banter can be confusing and alienating. Yet one of their biggest problems can be an inability to read their own emotional world, with difficulties in working out what they are feeling.

Symptoms of anxiety or depression, for example, can find expression in all sorts of other behavioural ways or as physical symptoms, which might not be immediately recognised as arising from an emotional problem.

But then, in 2013, with DSM-5, things changed. The categories of autism and all the related diagnoses (such as Asperger's) were coalesced into the same category under the rubric of ASD, or autism spectrum disorder. There were good reasons for doing this, in recognising that they were related neurodevelopmental disorders, but as Allen Frances said, 'Rule of thumb – if anything in a DSM can possibly be misused, it will be misused.'[12]

Once autism became conflated with milder, related conditions such as Asperger's, it was only a small step to start to include within the diagnostic net other individuals who were socially awkward, sensitive to environmental stimuli or struggled to conform to normal social expectations. Since then, we have seen a rise in the diagnosis of ASD to the extent that it is almost normal for a patient attending clinic to ask about it, just as Linda had. I considered what she had told me. Perhaps her social interactions had been less intuitive, more of an effort for her. And it is true to say that anxiety disorders commonly accompany ASD. Yet both anxiety and social awkwardness are common, and these difficulties did not seem to have held her back in life, in which she had spent a career having to communicate with people buying properties.

I found it hard to see how the diagnosis fit with what I knew of her, and it was difficult to know how to progress with this. A diagnosis is for life, and great care needs to be taken about making one based on mild symptoms that may be complicated by other problems such as anxiety. I wondered aloud how a diagnosis would help her. She told me that she was just curious, and when she thought about it, it might not make too much difference, except it might help to explain a few things about her life.

This was understandable and, if she wanted some help in navigating social interactions, reasonable too. But I felt cautious about referring Linda for a formal diagnosis when I had so many doubts about it, and my instinct was to continue to treat her anxiety, which would ultimately make a difference to how she felt about her life.

For children, a diagnosis of ASD really can make a difference in accessing the help they need at school and getting the right kind of support. There is also likely to be a cohort of undiagnosed adults who have never really had help to navigate the difficulties that their symptoms have caused them, or had their suffering acknowledged, or had a diagnosis that may, even late in the day, help them make sense of their lives. Paradoxically, I suspect that many autistic people with low support needs do not attend clinics for a diagnosis, because this is their normal.

Psychiatry is currently at a crossroads with neurodevelopmental disorders. We are trying to offer help to those who need it, and trying to retrospectively diagnose those adults whose diagnosis was missed. All the while, we are struggling to ensure that the boundaries are wide enough to encompass all the individuals who belong there and keep out those who don't. Yet somehow, along the way, the overlap of diagnoses with character traits previously considered as normal variations has become blurred. Perhaps our very definition of what is normal is changing at the same time. Yet it feels as if we, as a profession, are failing in our goal to differentiate the two. The consequence has been that neurodevelopmental services have been stretched beyond their capacity to cope, and what were once considered quite rare disorders have become commonplace. Time will tell if this has improved the overall mental health and well-being of the population. I hope on balance that it does, and that it leads to improved funding for services. Yet I am doubtful. My concern is that in our current desire to dispense and identify with a diagnostic label that explains some elements of our experience, we are starting to narrow the concept of normal, to limit our sense of who we are and how we live our lives, to reduce our conception of humanity in all its infinite, individual variations.

9

Personality and the Search for Normal

Personality is a fundamental concept in psychiatry. It is the base on which behaviours are built and aberrant actions understood. It can be a predisposing factor for more overt mental illness. And yet, personality and personality disorders have created a headache for psychiatry. Both are fluid, almost undefinable concepts that have increasingly taken hold in public discourse. Psychiatric name-calling invoking personality disorders ('he's such a narcissist . . . she's a real psychopath') is everywhere. But in the search for normal, what constitutes a normal personality, and how to reliably differentiate this from the abnormal and pathological, has so far proved a task beyond us. How much of a behaviour is too much? If your doctor checks your blood result twice, three times, are they being careful or obsessional? If you prefer others to make decisions for you, are you easy-going or do you have a dependent personality? If someone has an indifference to friendships, sexual relationships, praise or criticism, are they independent spirits or should that be counted as a schizoid personality?

We are hard-pressed to describe our own personalities. I routinely ask people to do this during consultations, and they struggle mightily. The eighteenth-century Scottish poet Robert Burns, in his poem 'To a Louse', spoke of the blind spot in understanding our own personalities ('O wad some Power the giftie gie us /

To see oursels as ithers see us!'). And which of us has not wished to see ourselves through other people's eyes and understand the impression that we make? Our interest in our own personalities, that staple of magazine 'personality quizzes' ('Relationship personality type! What's your ideal match? What type of person are you at work?!'), speaks to the uncertainty and insecurity in us all. We want some objective way of seeing ourselves, to understand how we fit into the world around us, or perhaps an explanation of why we don't.

The quizzes are – like horoscopes – generally based on what is commonly known as the 'Barnum effect', named after a nineteenth-century American circus owner who said, or was said to have said, that 'there is a sucker born every minute'. The Barnum effect has been described as the 'tendency for people to accept vague, ambiguous, and general statements as descriptive of their unique personalities'.[1] Statements like 'Outwardly you can seem confident, but inside can be full of doubt' or 'You are generally trusting of others, although once betrayed, it can be difficult to regain your trust' may feel personal to us, yet they are universal feelings, as are many of our thoughts and emotions. Is there anyone who doesn't feel a bit insecure inside? Or have a tendency to be a bit self-critical? Or like to see themselves as discerning thinkers, not accepting statements at face value but preferring evidence?

Psychologists have tried over many years to find that elixir, to distil down our specific personalities into the fewest number of attributes, like a unifying theory for personalities. One of the best known is commonly called the 'Big Five', thought to describe our five key personality factors, and is sometimes known by the acronym OCEAN.[2] Each factor exists on a spectrum, so that people may have some of the trait, a little of it or the inverse of it. The 'O' stands for openness, which describes people's openness to new experiences and ideas. It reflects something of the individual's intellectual curiosity and creativity. 'C' is conscientiousness, that quality of diligence, organisation, not being prone to erratic or impulsive behaviour. 'E' is extraversion. As you would expect, this describes people who are outgoing and engaging with a socially gregarious sort of personality. 'A' stands for agreeableness, which can be a spectrum of behaviour from supportive and sociable to self-centred and antagonistic. And finally, 'N' is for neuroticism, highlighting that overwrought, introspective, anxious kind of quality, as opposed to the stable and unflappable sort of individuals.

These types of scales suggest that people's personalities do seem to be stable over time, and perhaps they even tell us something about what the future might hold. One study, which took place over an unusually long, forty-five-year period, followed up university graduates in the US until retirement age.[3] The personality traits were correlated with a variety of outcomes. One of the most robust was that conscientiousness in younger years seemed to most closely predict how people would function later in life. Extraversion was correlated with income, which perhaps is a surprise, although it may have something to do with extroverts more easily making connections, networking and being easy to work with. Openness was associated with creativity, as well as, surprisingly, the use of psychiatric services.

The concept of personality disorders in psychiatry is, relatively speaking, a modern one. Even up to the nineteenth century, when doctors and philosophers talked about personality, they were referring to something different from that which we now understand.[4] Most of the early discussions about individual differences were framed in terms of temperaments rather than illnesses and disorders. People have always reacted differently to loss and adversity, frustration and struggle, risk and opportunity. Some are naturally cautious, some anxious, others selfish, obsessional, or perhaps cruel and unstable. Some have an optimistic temperament, or are natural leaders, whilst others struggle to leave their home, overwhelmed by the world and unable to make a decision for themselves. We each bring our own experiences, sometimes burdened with our ancestral history or a collective memory. This in turn provides the basis on which we see and understand the world around us and react to events.

Our temperaments or personalities can be changed by disease and injury. The story of Phineas Gage became well known because it provided one of the first clearly described links between our brain function and personality. Phineas Gage was a railroad worker in the US, who in 1848 suffered a freak occupational injury.[5] His job that day was to create a path for the railroad tracks, using dynamite to blast rocks that were in the way. To do this, a hole would be dug in the rock, gunpowder inserted into the hole, and then sand put over the gunpowder. The gunpowder would then be compacted down using a tamping iron over the sand. Once compacted, the gunpowder would be ignited and create an explosion, removing the rocks and obstacles to the railway path.

On this particular day, the sand was accidentally omitted, so when the tamping iron was dropped in the hole, it sparked the gunpowder, and the tamping iron exploded upwards, passing through Phineas Gage's cheek, up through his brain, and out of his skull at the top, landing some distance away ('high into the air, falling to the ground several rods behind him, where it was afterwards picked up by his men, smeared with blood and brain',[6] according to a contemporary, a physician named John Harlow). Amazingly, Gage survived the injury, despite considerable destruction done to the front part of his brain on the left side, in the area known as the frontal lobe.[5] Harlow further noted, 'His contractors, who regarded him as the most efficient and capable foreman in their employ previous to his injury, considered the change in his mind so marked that they could not give him his place again.'[6] He

was now 'fitful, irreverent, indulging at times in the grossest pro-
fanity (which was not previously his custom), manifesting but little
deference for his fellows, impatient of restraint or advice when
it conflicts with his desires, at times pertinaciously obstinate, yet
capricious and vacillating'.

Personality changes in relation to a variety of brain insults are
now well described. Brain tumours or injuries can cause changes
in personality, depending on where in the brain they are located.
People with damage in the frontal lobe can present similarly to
Phineas Gage, with a lack of social awareness, a coarsening of the
personality and a failure to take into account social norms and
standards of behaviour; others become apathetic or lack judgement – all these traits revealing in deficit some of the normal
functions of the frontal lobe in humans. Areas deeper in the brain,
such as the amygdala and hypothalamus, play a role in fear and
aggression.[7] These areas are part of a brain network known as
the limbic system, which broadly underlies emotional regulation.
Damage to these areas, depending on exactly where and by how
much, can lead to uncontrolled rage, placidity, changes in sexual
behaviour or propensity to addictions.[8]

For a time, people with epilepsy arising from their temporal
lobes were thought to have particular personality types,[9] which
became known as Geschwind syndrome. Their temperaments
were said to be characterised by low sex drive, a tendency towards
excessive writing, sometimes called hypergraphia, and what was
called 'religiosity', a kind of excessive piety.[10] I have seen these
traits from time to time in patients with epilepsy. Patients arrive
in the clinic with notebooks packed full of musings and notes. I
have seen individuals who previously considered themselves arch-
rationalists or atheists discovering a deep devotion to religion after
the epilepsy has begun. Yet tempting though it is to think that the
epileptic activity in a brain is driving personality, the notion of

a personality variant specific to epilepsy has been disputed[11] and probably discounted. It seems that the studies never really differentiated the effects of epilepsy on the personality from the wider effects of mental illness, which of course can affect anyone.

It was really over the course of the twentieth century that personality disorders emerged into something more recognisable to the current way we use the term. At first, it was the more extreme personality types that were described, commonly those that brought the individual into contact with the police or courts. A Royal Commission report[12] published in 1908 introduced the term 'moral imbeciles' to describe what we would now recognise as psychopathic (commonly called dissocial or antisocial) personalities. Moral imbeciles were defined as 'persons who from an early age display some mental defect coupled with strong vicious or criminal propensities on which punishment has little or no deterrent effect'.[12] The definition was similar to the one recommended to the Commission by the Royal College of Physicians, aside from one change. Instead of 'some mental defect', the Royal College had suggested 'and in spite of careful upbringing'. In other words, the physicians were trying to draw out the idea that there was not really any obvious mental defect in such individuals, and no particular reason why they should be born to one family and not another.

Today there are a number of defined personality disorders in psychiatric use, although many of the people with them do not end up in a consulting room. Their disorders may come across in odd, idiosyncratic behaviours, or perhaps as obsessional or nervy and anxious temperaments, but these people are not ill in the common use of the word. Personality disorders may render some vulnerability to mental illness, but in contrast, many people with mental health problems have entirely normal personalities. The latest version of DSM clusters personality disorders into three broad groups. The first group (cluster A) consists of those that contain elements of paranoia, or odd and unusual thinking, such as schizoid, paranoid or schizotypal personalities. The second, cluster B, groups those personality types more likely to be seen in an individual's public behaviours, such as antisocial, narcissistic, borderline or histrionic personality disorder. And the final group, cluster C, contains the more vulnerable and anxious sorts of personality – avoidant, dependent, obsessional. I have heard the clusters characterised, rather unkindly, as 'mad, bad and sad', although it does reflect something of the reality of the clusters. Yet the fact remains that most of these individuals are not ill in any normal sense of the word. They are variants of personality that can make navigating life harder.

There is increasingly a divergence in the way that psychiatrists and the public understand personality disorders. Psychiatrists have struggled with the concept of personality, something that evades clear-cut definition whilst being fundamental to what it means to be human. It is even harder with personality disorders to find a definition that separates those with and without in a way that is meaningful and therapeutic, particularly at the milder ends of behaviour. A great deal of humility and caution is needed. Yet personality disorders have been latched on to by the public as real, living entities with crisp boundaries. Words like narcissist, psychopath, passive-aggressive and borderline have entered the language and are used as a means of insulting or belittling someone. I also think they are used as a means of absolving oneself from any blame. If the other person is a narcissist or a psychopath, then surely they, and not us, are responsible for everything that happened next. The use of the terms starts to generate its own reality. Personality disorders start to be seen as belonging to people who have offended or upset us in some way.

The definition of antisocial personality disorder has been altered and revised over time, although it has always been recognisably similar to current definitions. The World Health Organization's International Classification of Diseases, ICD-10, published in 1992, and the one I have used for nearly all of my career, defined antisocial personality disorders as being characterised by a 'callous unconcern for the feelings of others'.[13] People with antisocial personalities are able to form relationships easily but lack the deeper feelings and connections that are the bedrock of any adult relationship. Maintaining relationships is therefore much more difficult than starting them. There is a low tolerance to frustration, and violence can be easily triggered. ICD-10 also adds that people with dissocial personalities have 'a marked proneness to blame others or to offer plausible rationalizations' for why they were not in the wrong when in a dispute or altercation.

There have been many screen portrayals reflecting this personality type. Begbie, the character in the Irvine Welsh novel *Trainspotting*, who was played in the film by Robert Carlyle, is an archetype. There is a scene when he spills his pint down his shirt whilst in a pub. It is entirely his fault. He has carelessly knocked his tray of full pint glasses of beer against someone else as he walks to his table, but somehow sees himself as the aggrieved party. His fury cannot be assuaged, and nor can his violence in the subsequent brawl. Ben Kingsley's character Don Logan in the movie *Sexy Beast* is another wonderful portrayal of dissocial personality disorder. Both characters straddle the boundary on the edge of the law, bringing to mind another ICD-10 descriptor, an 'incapacity to experience guilt or to profit from experience, particularly punishment', so that even prison sentences are not particularly effective in changing behaviour.

When I have met people with antisocial personalities, the thing that always strikes me, before I have even really got the interview under way, is how I feel around them. Generally speaking, the mood a conversation generates, the feeling it gives you, is always worth paying attention to, particularly so in a clinical context. Freud referred to this as countertransference, the feeling that an individual evokes in their doctor. It is a communication of a kind, if you want to interpret it that way. Something is being said, not necessarily in words but in the interaction, the body language, the tone, that indefinable feel of a conversation. People with psychopathy set me on edge. I find myself excessively cautious, wary, formally polite and correct.

I remember the conversation I had with someone fitting this personality type on a hospital ward. Kieran was around forty, and the referral came from the surgical ward where he was recovering from orthopaedic surgery. As best I could understand, his foot had been run over by a car whilst he was walking in the street late at night. Since admission to the ward, Kieran had been disruptive, and the referring team wanted to know if this was part of a treatable psychiatric condition. The referral was vague, with no clear pointers of what the diagnosis might be beyond him being 'disruptive' and 'rude', which to a psychiatrist could mean more or less anything.

At the bedside, Kieran was initially polite. I asked a little about the foot injury, but five minutes later had still not quite got to the bottom of why he had been walking in the street on the night of his injury. There was a pub, a fight, ending with him looking for his assailants after they had left the pub, which still didn't explain why he was in the middle of the road. He was far keener to talk about his current problems on the ward. He told me that the nurses would not let him sleep, because they kept wanting to measure his blood pressure and take observations. He said that the hospital food was an insult to him, that the staff were 'winding him up'. And now a visit from a psychiatrist. To his mind, he told me, he was the victim. He felt that his outbursts were justified. I found out later that day that one of the nurses was so unnerved by his threat to discover her home address that she had refused to attend to him.

On the one hand, the case he made was quite plausible. The food was poor and the frequent observations interrupted his sleep. And yet on the other hand, these were the standards of care that others were getting, none of whom were making specific and personal threats to staff members. Later in the consultation, Kieran told me of someone in his past who had also 'wound him up'. I noted the choice of words.

'What happened? To the person winding you up.'

'He's on the wrong side of the grass.'

It was delivered in a self-satisfied way, seemingly as a warning that he was not to be messed with. I wasn't sure if I believed him, but he wouldn't give me any other details, and there was nowhere really to go with it. When I asked more about it, he cut across me, 'Now you're starting to wind me up.'

Hospitals can be stressful places, and sometimes people can act out of character there, but Kieran's behaviour could not easily be put down to the stress of it all. I was aware in the moment of my feelings and reactions. I felt threatened and uneasy, and I began to wonder if I would become the focus of his ire for asking a lot of personal and intrusive questions. In an attempt to diffuse the unpleasantness of future hard feelings, I was overly courteous, almost ingratiating.

There was little I could offer from the point of view of treating Kieran's personality. And from the ward's perspective, there were not going to be any easy ways to manage this situation, apart from trying to agree a behavioural contract with the patient. Behavioural contracts are agreements that set out which patient behaviours will be tolerated and not tolerated, and what the outcome might be for breaching the contract. These sometimes include a formal warning to the patient, discharge from the hospital or transfer to a different hospital. But deep down I knew it wouldn't work. They are rarely, if ever, enforced, and once that happens, then you've lost any leverage you had.

People with antisocial personality disorders are more commonly seen in forensic psychiatry, that branch of psychiatry where mental health intersects with the law. Antisocial behaviour often brings individuals into conflict with others, or to the attention of the police, and from there to psychiatry. Our ability as psychiatrists to make meaningful changes to such personality disorders though is very much a work in progress.

Another common type of personality is known as borderline personality disorder (sometimes called emotionally unstable personality disorder). It was described in the late 1930s by the psychoanalyst Adolf Stern,[14] and the name has caused confusion ever since its inception, as it appears to suggest a personality that is just beyond the boundary of normal. In fact, it was initially named 'borderline' because it was conceptualised as being on the borderline of psychosis and neurosis, although subsequent studies found no relationship between this disorder and psychotic illnesses like schizophrenia. The symptoms of borderline personality disorder can be hard to describe and are hard to relate to because, unlike illnesses such as depression, they involve experiences that many people won't have ever had, even in a diluted form, such as persistent feelings of emptiness inside, or lacking a real sense of who one is. Fear of abandonment in threatened or actual relationship breakdowns can be overwhelming, and one of the means of coping with these intense emotions can be self-harm. In this respect, feeling the pain or seeing the blood after self-harm is cathartic. 'At least,' such patients will tell me, 'I am feeling something.'

Most of the time, these acts of self-harm do not come to medical attention. Yet there is undoubtedly a higher risk of suicide and suicidal behaviours in people with borderline personality disorder.[15, 16] And there are many behaviours that fall somewhere between self-harm and suicide attempts, a certain kind of reckless-ness, often an uncertainty within the individual themselves, about what the expected or desired outcome is. Again, I return to my own emotional reaction after a consultation with someone with this personality type. It is one of doubt. There is a lingering uncer-tainty that I carry throughout my day. I feel a mix of emotions, a cloud of agitated sadness and unease, often a kind of helplessness. This feeling is probably only an echo of what the individual is feeling, which must be horribly difficult and lonely.

Manny was a young man whom I saw on many occasions over a period of around six months who gave me exactly this feel-ing. He had long-standing surgical problems related to a traumatic injury sustained some years prior, for which he'd had many oper-ations, and was frequently readmitted for treatment of infections or revisions of previous operations. I met him for the first time on a hospital ward. He wanted to take his own discharge, but the doctors were concerned that in doing so, he would be putting his health at significant risk. They wanted to know if mental illness may be impairing his judgement.

It was a bright summer afternoon, and when I arrived on the ward, I found Manny lying in his hospital bed, thin blue curtains pulled around for privacy. He was in the corner, curled up facing the wall with his back to the room. A fan in the recess by the window blew warm air at us, rattling away noisily as it turned.

'Hello, I'm Dr Santhouse, one of the psychiatry doctors. I've heard you want to go home, but the doctors think you need to stay in hospital. Could I ask you some more about that?'

Manny did not turn round to look at me. He just lay there on the bed, so I carried on talking to his back as though I hadn't noticed, whilst he lay there mute. After around ten minutes of this, he suddenly sat up, told me that he had decided he liked me, and carried on with the consultation as if nothing had happened.

Manny's story was of a broken home, an unhappy school career and now living alone in a council flat with little to occupy his time. He had siblings that he had only intermittent contact with, and whom I only met once. In his hospital gown, Manny revealed a mass of scars up and down both arms, and he told me of many other episodes of self-harm over the years. These had come in a variety of ways, often overdoses, or not taking his diabetic medication and letting his blood sugars run out of control. These had led him into psychiatric care over recent years, with psychological therapies and support, but little that had made a meaningful change in his way of seeing the world. He spoke of a feeling of futility, struggling to make any sense of life. There was a chronic and pervasive boredom, with no ambitions, no notion of what he was about or who he really was. He found it hard to articulate but told me that he didn't think he was cut out for this world. Relationships were few and far between. He would get too attached and then bombard his partner with anxious and increasingly desperate messages, accelerating the outcome he feared the most – of being abandoned. We finally got round to talking about the issue at hand. He told me that once he took his own discharge, he wasn't sure what he would do. I asked if his uncertainty included whether he would attend the ward regularly for treatment, or would he neglect his health and cause harm this way, perhaps even endangering his life.

'I can't answer that,' he said, smiling.

'Why not?'

'Because I don't know what I'll do.'

'Well, if you were in my position, looking after you, what would you do?'

'That's up to you, isn't it?'

I felt trapped. On the one hand, there was always going to be a risk if he went home. His personality, at least at this stage of his life, meant that he was overall at much higher risk of coming to harm than the rest of the population. But by forcing the issue, detaining him on the ward, I feared that the situation would start to escalate to become unpleasantly coercive, and set up a dynamic that would destroy his relationship with the medical profession. Manny knew my dilemma, and for a moment I was in his world, of uncertainty, anxiety, indecision. I think, at least subconsciously, it was where he wanted me. Eventually, and with some misgivings, I decided that Manny did not have a mental illness sufficient to impair his judgement and that he could take his own discharge if he wanted to.

I went back to my office, checked some emails, but couldn't quite settle. I remembered when I was a junior doctor, one of the senior consultants telling me that what you got paid for as a consultant was not the large number of straightforward decisions but the occasional very difficult one. This was one of them. With a sinking heart, I called the ward to find out what had happened to Manny. The charge nurse told me he had decided to stay and complete his treatment. The previous couple of hours of worry had been for nothing.

I came to like Manny over the time I got to know him, but a call from the ward whenever he was readmitted nearly always presented me with a similar problem. Sometimes he would be bright and friendly, at others would refuse to talk to me, but never was he able to give the reassurance that I sought when it came to his safety. I just had to live with it – and of course, in a more meaningful way, so did he. And things continued like this until his care was transferred to another hospital for follow-up, once his physical health problems had largely resolved. I didn't see him after that, although I did once see his new psychiatry consultant around a year later. We discussed Manny's care, and my colleague told me he'd had a similar experience. The ambition of his treating team was harm reduction and support. Nobody thought that the concept of cure was a realistic goal, something that can be very difficult to achieve when personality disorders are as severe as Manny's.

Perhaps the most well-known personality disorder is one that is rarely seen clinically – or at least not as the main reason for attending. This is because, for the most part, people who have the features associated with narcissistic personality disorder do not typically see themselves as needing help. Perhaps this is why people seem so ready to diagnose it for them. Accusations of narcissism are common on social media platforms, an almost meaningless put-down for someone whose behaviour you disagree with. Questionnaires appear online asking if your boss or ex-partner is a secret narcissist, along with checklists revealing how to 'spot a narcissist'. If there were a league table of modern diagnoses that have become detached from any meaningful clinical sense, narcissism would be a strong contender for one of the top places.

The ICD-10 understood narcissistic personality disorder as 'an enduring pattern of grandiose beliefs and arrogant behavior together with an overwhelming need for admiration and a lack of empathy for (and even exploitation of) others'.[17] Some people with narcissism experience low self-esteem and sensitivity to criticism.[18] One might speculate that grandiose and arrogant behaviours may act as a defence, as a way of managing this vulnerability.

During the 2016 US presidential election and since then, a lot was spoken of Donald Trump's apparent narcissism. One US clinician, described as a 'leading psychiatrist', was reported as saying that Trump had narcissistic personality disorder. 'Donald Trump . . . suffers from extremely severe mental disorders, which render him incapable of attending to any issue beyond his own personal need for adulation. The mental condition he suffers most from is formally known as a severe instance of "narcissistic personality disorder".'[19]

I was troubled by this. There seemed to be a rash of therapists and others saying similar things, people who had never met Donald Trump. There was a rule in the US about psychiatrists not diagnosing mental health problems without making a proper assessment of the individual, known as the Goldwater rule.[20] It was eminently sensible because, particularly for personality disorders, a thorough assessment is always necessary. Making a judgement on someone's personality is a serious business, with many traps for the unwary. For a start, the public persona may not match the private thoughts or behaviours of the individual, and close family and friends may be able to give a longitudinal and different perspective. These sources of information are not, of course, usually available to armchair analysts, no matter how experienced. Yet, it was argued,[20] in the rush to judge Donald Trump's personality, the Goldwater rule was applied only to psychiatrists, and not to psychologists, whose ethical rules did not preclude such speculation. One paper proposed that there were 'select cases in which psychological scientists with suitable expertise may harbor a "duty to inform", allowing them to offer informed opinions concerning public figures' mental health with appropriate caveats'.[20]

Readers, as well as the wider press, did not focus on the caveats. They saw only that a public figure had been diagnosed with narcissistic personality disorder. But what, I wondered, was this 'duty to inform' the public about? What were the public meant to do with this new information? And how did this add to what they could already see with their own eyes? Donald Trump's personal shortcomings were hardly a secret. Furthermore, there was nothing therapeutic in making a diagnosis of personality disorder for the individual 'diagnosed'. As clinicians, we are supposed to make a diagnosis as the basis for providing treatment, not merely for our own, or public, interest. And finally, how were we able to know that a psychologist's own biases had not influenced their

diagnosis from afar and clouded their objectivity? A similar accusation was levelled by a British psychiatrist towards Boris
Johnson in the run-up to the UK general election in 2019 – that
he had a personality disorder which rendered him unfit for office
– which led me to one of the very few arguments I have ever had
on X/Twitter. In both cases, such comments felt to me little more
than psychiatric name-calling, a type of character assassination
under the cloak of righteousness and with a veneer of science to
give it respectability.

I would maintain that no psychologist or psychiatrist should
express a public opinion on the presence of a personality disorder
based only on someone's public persona and pronouncements. I
have no idea whether either Donald Trump or Boris Johnson has
a personality disorder, and I think the speculation itself is unfair.
The public know enough about each of them to form a view as to
whether they would like them to be president or prime minister,
and that is as much as anyone needs to know.

Away from the rarefied echelons of politics, the management of
people's personalities in the real world of medical care can cause
a great deal of uncertainty. One example in which a psychiatric judgement upon personality carried significant weight both
legally and medically was in the case of 'C', a fifty-year-old woman
whose case came before the Court of Protection in 2015.[21] This
was not someone whom I had met. I remember learning about
the case for the first time when I read about it in the press, where
it received widespread coverage. It seemed to strike a nerve with
the public. The case concerned C's capacity to accept or refuse
life-saving medical treatment following an overdose. The court
heard that in the lead-up to the overdose, C had gone to her
daughter's house and asked for some expensive champagne, which
she later drank along with a large number of tablets. The overdose was not quite enough to kill her, but it did cause significant

liver damage, which in turn stopped her kidneys from working, meaning that she needed dialysis to keep her alive. After a time, C decided that she didn't want dialysis, even though her liver had by now recovered, and her kidneys were in time expected to recover to the point that she would no longer require dialysis.

The months leading up to the overdose had not been easy for C. She'd had breast cancer in 2014, followed by lumpectomy and radiotherapy in the first half of 2015. Soon after the cancer treatment had concluded, there had been what the court described as the 'acrimonious breakdown of a long term relationship'. She'd lost her home, her business and her financial security and had incurred significant debt. In the context of this relationship breakup, there was an incident that led to her arrest and criminal charges. It was following this that C had decided to take an overdose of paracetamol tablets along with the champagne.

At the heart of the court's decision was the impact of C's personality on her decision-making capacity. The judge needed to decide whether her personality affected her ability to adequately weigh up the risks and benefits of either having treatment or withdrawing from treatment, and to come to a sound decision about whether to continue or withdraw from dialysis.

Drawing on testimony from many people who knew her, a picture of C's personality emerged. The judgement of the case stated, 'C has led a life characterised by impulsive and self-centred decision making without guilt or regret. C has had four marriages and a number of affairs and has, it is said, spent the money of her husbands and lovers recklessly before moving on when things got difficult or the money ran out. She has, by their account, been an entirely reluctant and at times completely indifferent mother to her three caring daughters.'[21]

C's daughter concurred with this view, saying, 'My mother's values, and the choices that she made have always been based on looks (hers and other people's), money, and living (at all costs) what she called her "*sparkly*" lifestyle . . . her life was, from her point of view, a life well lived. I have never known her express regret, or really to take responsibility for anything, including the choices she has made.'[21]

Now that the prospect of a life without sparkle was looming, as age and all the pleasures and pains associated with it were becoming a reality, C decided that she did not want to have the dialysis, even if it was to be temporary, and even if not doing so led to her death. To her, there was no upside to ageing, or being poor, or having an unattractive figure. Thoughts of her family did not deter her. The court had noted that she had previously been angry to discover that her daughter was pregnant, since that would make her a grandmother and 'past her sell-by date'.

It was speculated in court that C's strongly held and unconventional opinions may have reflected a personality disorder, at one stage considered as a possible histrionic personality disorder. Elsewhere, it was considered that her behaviour might be explained by narcissistic personality disorder. But as one of the psychiatrists assisting the court pointed out, 'there are no validated tools in this area to ascertain a baseline of "normal" in the context of diagnosing personality problems'. And whilst the judge acknowledged that C's decision would be seen by many as unwise, and by some as immoral, C had her own value system, one accepted by the judge as valid, in which she made a whole different set of calculations about the value of her life. She was judged to have capacity to refuse dialysis.[21]

This is the sort of case that exposes the boundaries of personalities and personality disorders. How does one try to understand a decision like C's? What calculation makes death preferable to living? Just because C saw things entirely differently from many other people, is that the only basis on which we would say her personality was disordered? Or could her worldview be accepted as unconventional but normal?

But the case also highlights another problem with personality disorders, and that is – as the psychiatrist said in court – the difficulty of accurate diagnosis. In past versions of DSM, personality disorders tended to have overlapping criteria, which made it difficult to justify them as discrete diagnostic entities. One study showed that 54% of patients diagnosed with one personality disorder, using the criteria at that time, would have qualified for a diagnosis of more than one personality disorder.[22]

This lack of specificity between different personality disorders led to some changes in the most recent iteration of DSM, which holds that there are ten distinct and diagnosable personality types.[22] But DSM-5 also developed a hybrid model, which means that as well as being able to diagnose personality disorders (antisocial, borderline, obsessional, etc.) as discrete entities, it is also possible to describe personalities on a spectrum using a number of personality descriptors. The World Health Organization, in its latest International Classification of Diseases (ICD-11), has now moved fully over to this dimensional model as a way of describing personality disorders. In ICD-11, each person can be scored on each of five domains (negativity, detachment, disinhibition, dissociality and anankastia (obsessionality/perfectionism)), and the personality disorder can be mild, moderate or severe.[23]

Whilst dimensional descriptions are undoubtedly a more accurate way of describing someone, they are not always helpful to a clinician when trying to communicate something about a patient. By way of analogy, many human characteristics exist on a dimension, for example, blood pressure and height. It may be more accurate to give the exact reading, for example, 165/110, or six feet two inches, but sometimes it communicates more to say that the person is hypertensive or tall. And therein lies the dilemma in psychiatry. Do we prefer the more descriptive dimensions of personality, measured on a number of different domains (for example, how negative is this person? How obsessional? Do they have elements of dissocial behaviour? Disinhibition?) and give a comprehensive and accurate description, albeit wordier and more complicated? Or do we sacrifice some of the accuracy for a crisper way of communicating a diagnosis at the expense of losing some of the detail? The consensus is shifting to the former, more descriptive approach. It's more accurate and fairer, but my prediction is that it won't be used much by practising clinicians. It is cumbersome, time-consuming and, most importantly, does not easily convey meaning in the way that a diagnostic label would.

The understanding of personality disorders is constantly evolving, although it is not clear that it is advancing. We seem to be describing a reality that everyone sort of understands, but nobody can quite put their finger on. People with personality disorders often struggle to make their way in the world, and these disorders, as ICD-11 expresses it, are 'nearly always associated with considerable personal and social disruption'.[24] The origins of personality disorders are varied and inconsistent. Some personality disorders, such as paranoid personality, can be seen in descriptions from ancient Greece; others derive from clinical observation. Some, such as compulsive personalities, have their roots in psychodynamic theory (for example, Freud's anal retentives), and others are the result of committee consensus.[4] In 1999, the UK government even invented one of its own, 'dangerous severe personality disorder',[25,26] in an attempt to identify and treat people with personality disorders who were considered at high risk of committing serious criminal offences. Yet it was ultimately a project that ran aground. It proved almost impossible to reliably measure the severity of personality disorders, and it was hard to predict the criminal risk. The disorder was quietly dropped, and has since been merged into the offender personality disorder pathway,[27] a service for people whose personality disorder is linked to criminal offending.

I have also wondered about how we have collectively limited the number of personality types we can diagnose. If the ultimate definition of personality disorders is that they are enduring patterns of behaviour that bring the sufferer into conflict with society, or impair their progress in areas of their life, what about other behaviours? What of a man who neglects his family because of a drive to spend all his time at the office? His behaviour can cause marital disharmony, impact on the children, get in the way of holidays and family outings. It seems like an entirely unreasonable behaviour, but the workaholic has no formal personality disorder. Or how about the woman whose personality and self-esteem become based around lip fillers, botox, false eyelashes and her figure? This does not seem like a healthy way to live either. So when do we define these as a problem, as some form of mental health disorder that requires treatment?

Labels of personality disorder are conveying something real, if hard to grasp. We know they can increase vulnerability to mental illness and suicide, and cause distress to both those suffering and people around them. It's just that in the absence of any objective way of diagnosing them, no blood tests or brain scans, we can struggle to give them the precision we want and explain exactly what we mean.

Another problem with these diagnostic labels is the impact they have on the individuals diagnosed. A label seems to imply, even if it was not the intention, that they are fundamentally flawed individuals – they don't just have a problem; they are a problem. One study showed that, even within psychiatry, if someone had a personality disorder label, they were seen by psychiatrists as annoying, manipulative and less deserving of care.[28] The authors of the study even suggested the concept of personality disorder be abandoned. The diagnosis still has the power to hurt and offend. It is not the type of diagnosis that people want to own, despite all the other work done in reducing mental health stigma. And perhaps this is why it is still used as an insult, both casually as a character assassination in a gossipy conversation with a friend and to traduce the reputation of a celebrity or politician. I often caution medical students that recognising the features of a personality disorder in someone you know does not mean that you should tell them. Maybe for this reason alone, a dimensional classification, where the personality is described without giving it a label, is kinder. Yet kindness and clinical utility are not the same thing. We just can't seem to square the circle. In a distant future, maybe our thoughts and behaviours will be visible to scanners as they travel through individual neurones in our brain. Perhaps we will point at the picture the scanner produces and say things like, 'There's a dependent personality disorder if I ever saw one.' Until then, defining personality is like having a duvet that's too short – however you position it, something is always sticking out.

10

Sex, Sexuality, Love and Gender

There can't be many areas of daily life where the insertion of psychiatry has been as contentious as those of sex, love and gender. It is hard to think of a single topic that is more influenced by the shifting sands of societal norms and acceptability. There is also no subject more personal to the core of an individual's identity. Predictably then, passionate arguments are made on every side of the debate. To make matters worse, debates are commonly uninformed by evidence, or at least not good-quality evidence, which makes them more a matter of opinion than a quest for scientific truth.

Homosexuality is probably the paradigm of how to mismanage a psychiatric diagnosis. It is a lesson in prejudice dressed up as scientific reason, only sustainable by a societal system that supported it.

When I was a trainee in psychiatry almost thirty years ago, I was handed a booklet on how to take a history. A psychiatric history is based around a loose structure, with plenty of latitude to follow up on whatever line of enquiry seems relevant. As you would expect, a significant amount of time within the history is expended on the main issue at hand, namely why the individual is consulting with you in the first place. Relevant to that is their past medical history, and whether or not the reason they are seeing you now is a recurrence of an old problem. If it is, you need to know what has been tried before and whether it helped. By the end of this discussion, you will have a pretty good idea of what is going on, and a diagnosis will often start to emerge. Yet no psychiatrist would be able to reach a proper conclusion without an understanding of the individual's personal history, a narrative of all the milestones of their life. It includes where they were born, their early childhood, the atmosphere at home as they were growing up, their experience of school, higher education, employment, relationships. Without a context for their problems, it can be hard to make sense of why they may have developed, or what sort of treatments might help.

The booklet walked the trainee through the main bullet points, but also suggested some other prompts. One of them, a question to female patients, was their age at menarche. It struck me even then as strangely archaic. I am aware of some research suggesting that early menarche may predispose to depression, but the question seemed unnecessarily intrusive, and if there was no way of making use of the answer, what was the point in asking the question? Another prompt was to ask about masturbation, and again, whatever one's views on the practice and morality of it, there are not many people who fear going blind because of it, nor I suspect feel the same moral conflicts about it as may have been the case in a more religious age. I would not now ask about masturbation at a consultation unless it was directly relevant to why the patient is attending, and over the years it has rarely come up.

Homosexuality is something I used to ask about far more routinely than I do today. Whilst for many people who are gay, it can still be a significant issue, both within families and in the workplace, overall it does not have the same impact on someone's mental health as it did a generation ago. Back then, being gay was routinely hidden away, 'coming out' could destroy families and careers, and casual homophobia was so commonplace that it was the punchline of many jokes. Today, it is largely acknowledged as another form of normal sexuality.

Homosexuality has been around for as long as humanity, and attitudes around it have reflected the different cultures over time. Some were religious and oppressive, some more permissive, but it was only in 1952, with the introduction of DSM-I, that homosexuality was classified as a diagnosis. As Drescher sets out, in an outstanding review article on psychiatry and homosexuality, the origin of this decision to consider homosexuality as a psychiatric illness was conceived in the late nineteenth century,[1] driven by the science of the time, based on Darwinian theory. This held that the purpose of sex was procreation and the perpetuation of the species. Through this lens, homosexuality was a form of degeneracy. It went against nature and, in so doing, must be a pathology, something broken within the human being. In the thinking of the time, this defect would count as a diagnosis. There was no getting away from it. Even if it could be shown that homosexuality is something one was born with, the individual was not exonerated – it would then simply be a congenital disease.

In this way, the trap was set. All acts of sex, including masturbation, that did not lead to the perpetuation of humanity were viewed as symptoms of a disease rather than simply as a behaviour. Undoubtedly, religious opinions had also become incorporated into this perspective of homosexuality, as well as the more censorious and intolerant view of difference that reflected the time in which this decision was taken.

It is hard to think of a more pernicious stance to take against a community already facing adversity and shame. The consequences were manifold. Firstly, the assertion that homosexuals were suffering from a form of mental illness logically led to attempts to cure them of their affliction. This approach is within the memory of some of my mentors in psychiatry. One of the treatments of homosexuality was to use a form of behavioural conditioning. The idea was that the subject needed to associate homosexuality with something unpleasant and aversive to put them off it. So, for example, a man would be shown pictures of naked men, which would be paired with a small electric shock applied to the body. The belief was that after a while, once the treatment was completed, even seeing a naked man would be associated in the recesses of the mind with something unpleasant happening, and in this way subconsciously put them off their attraction to other men. By contrast, during the treatment, pictures of the opposite sex would be shown in the absence of pain, in the hope that this connection between the opposite sex and relief from unpleasant feelings would be cemented in the mind of the unfortunate individual. Sometimes people agreed to have such treatment because of the social pressures brought to bear on them. Sometimes people would submit to the procedure to quell internalised shame, or simply because of a wish just to 'be normal' and belong in mainstream society. Others would agree to undergo treatment as an alternative to prison, in the days when homosexuality was still a criminal offence.[2]

Psychotherapy also had something to say about homosexuality. The classical Freudian interpretation was that homosexuality was 'arrested development', a normal and universal stage of human development in which the individual had simply got stuck.[3] All humans, so the theory went, passed through a stage of same-sex attraction, and some people simply didn't emerge to the other side. Freud himself was quite comfortable with homosexuality and the contributions of homosexual people to society. He did not appear to consider that homosexuality was a problem or believe that attempts to treat it were likely to work.[1]

The psychotherapy successors to Freud, though, were less circumspect in their views. Homosexuality was pathologised as an abnormal state of being. Gay men were more feminine, and gay women more masculine, or with both having some phobic avoidance of the opposite sex, or they were incapable of forming lasting relationships, or depressed, or any number of other speculative deficiencies to account for their state.[3] Psychoanalytic treatments were advanced for its cure. These aimed to understand the 'pathology' that had led to the state of homosexuality and, in understanding this, to effect a cure. The fact that openly gay or lesbian people were barred from enrolling in most psychoanalytic training[3] no doubt perpetuated the treatment of homosexuality as an illness.

As well as these treatments and aversion therapy, some people were subjected to chemical treatment, as in the shameful case of Alan Turing. Despite being credited with saving millions of lives in World War Two, because of his homosexuality, in 1952 he was convicted of gross indecency, and chose treatment with a synthetic oestrogen (with the effects including loss of libido and breast growth) rather than prison.[4]

It can be observed frequently in medicine throughout the ages that enthusiastic supporters of a treatment can influence practice, at least for a time, before the weight of evidence starts to catch up with them. But for a time at least, treatments for homosexuality continued, their effectiveness often decided by those people carrying them out.[3] Problems were compounded by the fact that treatments for homosexuality were not standardised, making it difficult to be sure what was improving or what to attribute any changes to. It would also not be too fanciful to suppose that treated patients lied about whether treatment had worked, for understandable reasons.

So how did those who were treated feel about their treatment? As you might expect, follow-up studies showed that they were distressed by what had happened to them.[2] The treatments tended to increase their sense of isolation and shame, perhaps by highlighting their difference from the mainstream and the unacceptability of their sexual impulses. It is probably superfluous to add that the treatments did not work, simply causing a lot of misery along the way.

Homosexuality remained a criminal offence in the UK until 1967. It seems strange now, to modern sensibilities, that the sexual preferences of the populace were the government's business or had anything to do with the criminal justice system. When I was growing up in the UK in the 1970s and 1980s, attitudes towards gay people were still only tentatively recovering. I didn't know many people who were openly homosexual at school, and the ones who were didn't talk about it. My first conversation with someone who was 'out' took place in my first year at university. But whilst he was 'out' at university, at home he led a different life. His father had assured him that if any of his children were gay, they would no longer be welcome at home. It was whilst we were at university that the UK government introduced Section 28, the legislation that made the promotion of same-sex relationships illegal,[5] and was intended to include schools, amongst other places. The late 1980s was also the time of HIV and AIDS, which at that stage was pretty much a death sentence for those who caught the virus. The virus was initially far more common amongst homosexual people, and it was not long before comments were made that the virus was a divine punishment for immorality. Newspapers referred to AIDS as the 'gay plague'. The chief constable of Manchester, where I grew up, spoke of homosexuals having brought AIDS upon themselves, since they were 'swirling around in a cesspit of their own making'.[6]

Given the societal norms that operated back then, it is perhaps not surprising that homosexual people had higher rates of mental health problems. Homosexuality was never a mental illness, any more than handedness and eye colour are, but by defining it as such, we created a lot of actual mental health problems along the way.

Homosexuality as a diagnosis was removed from DSM in 1973 after a vote, although this was not quite the end of the story.[1] Subsequent editions of DSM allowed for a diagnosis to be made if someone was unhappy with their homosexuality, until it became clear that this too was unsustainable. If being unhappy with personal characteristics could qualify you for a diagnosis, it would need to include a whole lot more than homosexuality. The final full stop, when the whole topic was dropped by DSM, was not until 1987.

The discussion about sexuality leads on to perhaps one of the most contentious of current public debates, that of gender and gender identity. I have hesitated even to introduce the topic, because it is hard to find a good-faith discussion about it. I am reminded of hearing an American guest on the radio, aware that the topic under discussion was inherently divisive. He likened it to the third rail on the New York subway – touch it and you're dead. And so it is with this, where views are all too frequently distorted or taken out of context, and contrary views are not to be expressed. It is common to hear of complaints made to employers or regulators so that the originator of the dissenting opinion can be disciplined or silenced.

Gender issues didn't really enter my professional consciousness in any meaningful, clinical way until around the early 2000s. I had seen patients before with issues relating to gender, but as isolated and unusual cases. These patients were not well understood and perhaps even pitied. One of the earliest individuals I recall had undergone gender reassignment surgery, and after a while had realised that it was a mistake and had undergone procedures to try to reverse the surgery to return to his original state. The gender issues were not the direct reason for me seeing him, but neither were they unconnected from his mood symptoms. The case stuck in my mind though, and I wondered about the quality of the assessment that had given the green light to the original surgery. I also wondered about the mental anguish that the patient must have gone through that ended in him having unnecessary operations. I sensed from my discussion with the patient that understanding and sympathy for his predicament were in short supply. Aside from the diagnosis, unusually for me, I remember surprisingly little about the patient. In place of the whole colourful picture of a life lived, my memory is just a mood, an emotion, a pall of sadness. He seemed alone and adrift, with a problem that nobody was able to help him with. Where were his family and friends? He had somehow ended up in a medical system that was not equipped to help him with his difficulties, but it would have to do – there was really nowhere else for him to go.

It was a couple of years later, in that same morning clinic, that a young man came to see me. He was a university student whose main clinical problem was related to unexplained pain. I took a careful history, asking about mood, anxiety, general mental health, personality and past medical history. I asked about his personal life and relationships, and this is when the consultation began to go off on a tangent. He told me that he did not feel particularly one gender or another, and I asked some more about what he meant. It was my first introduction to terms like 'cis,' 'trans' and 'gender-fluid', which are now part of common discourse but were back then rather niche terms, except at universities, where there was something of a revolution taking place. At first, I was not quite sure how or whether these terms related to sexual preference. The consultation by now had become somehow reversed, as the patient began to explain the terms to me, and I sat there taking notes, intending to look the terms up after the appointment. Whilst he explained everything with patience, I still wasn't sure I had entirely got things clear in my mind.

It was only a short time later that I found myself back in my old college for my thirty-year reunion. It was whilst I was strolling to dinner, in a dinner suit I hadn't worn since university that barely buttoned up at the waist, that I noticed posters petitioning the college to provide non-gendered toilets. It stopped me in my tracks. I hadn't known anyone either during my childhood or whilst at university for whom this might have been an issue. Yet this was twice now in the space of a couple of months that I had come across issues of gender raised by university students. As is often the case of social or political movements arising from universities, I felt it portended a change in social attitudes, or something that at the very least would change the conversation.

What is evident in contemporary society is the substantial increase over recent years in the number of people identifying as transgender. Studies in the US have shown an increase particularly amongst the younger adult population.[7] The same increase can also be seen in Europe and the Antipodes.[8] From the UK perspective, the national census of 2021 asked about gender identity in people over the age of sixteen.[9] Among the people surveyed, 93.5% said that their identity was the same as that at birth, 6% did not answer the question and 0.5%, or 262,000 people, stated that their gender was different from their sex assigned at birth. Even if everyone who declined to answer the question identifies with their gender at birth, over a quarter of a million people in the UK do not, which is still a substantial number. The number of people presenting to clinics for help or treatment with gender identity disorders has skyrocketed. The Gender Identity Development Service in the NHS, a service for young people, recorded 210 referrals to their service in 2011–12. A decade later, for the year 2021–22, there were 3,585 recorded referrals, a seventeen-fold increase in ten years.[10]

The reason for the increase in the number of transgender individuals worldwide is not clear, but it does need to be thought about and, if possible, explained. I would imagine part of the reason is that people who had previously felt ashamed by their gender identity no longer feel that they need to hide themselves away. Instead of retreat and shame, there is something more positive in owning the reality of who they are.

For some young people, part of the explanation may be in them exploring their own identity, as adolescents have done since the beginning of time. There seems to be far less peer disapproval of them alighting on a new, transgender identity, wearing it for a while to see if it fits, and shrugging it off without feeling as if this is a difficult or humiliating climbdown. This is a significant generational change. Previously, when someone had come out as gay, it was often preceded by years of agonising, hesitation and indecision. Now, identity change is more acceptable and, whilst not easy, there is undoubtedly less difficulty in doing so, and a fluidity that was once lacking.

The debate has centred around what adults should do about this, how parents, schools or medical services should respond, and here there has been near total paralysis. The topic has become too highly charged. There are those who have advocated a rigid rejection of the very idea of transgender and, by contrast, those who have encouraged automatic acceptance and affirmation. The Royal College of Psychiatrists recommended a neutral approach, advocating for further research. Whilst sensible in many ways, it was not always helpful to clinicians. More recently though, the Cass report reviewed gender identity services for children and young people in the UK and it made for uncomfortable reading.

Writing in the *BMJ*, the report's author, Hilary Cass, said that current practice has been 'built on shaky foundations' and that 'the majority of clinical guidelines have not followed the international standards for guideline development'.[11] Another article in the same edition of the *BMJ* spelt out the problem more starkly: 'The evidence base for interventions in gender medicine is threadbare, whichever research question you wish to consider – from social transition to hormone treatment.'[12]

My own clinical experience with gender identity disorders has been varied. Undoubtedly, it is something that I, and other psychiatrists, are seeing a great deal more often. At a recent clinic appointment, the individual I saw was a transgender man, which is to say that he had been born female and made the transition to male. As I collected him from the waiting room, I noticed perhaps something slightly more feminine about the features, but since the referral letter had said that he was male, and the referral related to persistent fatigue, I didn't give it much thought. It was only two-thirds of the way through the consultation that it came up, entirely tangentially to the problem with which he had presented. I think the biggest issue for the patient was not about gender, since that had been addressed and dealt with, but rather about other people's attitudes. They seemed sure that secretly he had some unresolved psychodynamic conflict to explain the fatigue, and the doctors kept wanting to pursue that route rather than the more standard medical path. I explored this with him a little before concluding that there really was no mileage in the trans discussion and getting on with the job in hand. In the end, the transgender aspect was only a footnote in the clinic letter, and I didn't feel the fatigue had anything to do with the transition that he had been through.

I have had other consultations where gender identity has been front and centre of the reason for referral. I remember seeing Seda in the clinic, a name chosen by the patient to reflect what she told me was the spirit of the forest. At the point when we met, the question of preferred pronouns had not been settled and Seda didn't mind she/her, so I followed her lead. Whilst I had understood, based on the referral, that the clinical problem would be a fairly straightforward anxiety disorder, once she arrived, it was clear that her issues were far more nuanced and complex. Her anxiety, she told me, was being caused by a deep unhappiness with her gender (female) and her difficulty in convincing the medical profession to accept this. She had come to get a psychiatric endorsement so that she could start hormone treatment. We began to talk, and she told me that she had always struggled to understand her feelings and did not have a strong sense of who she was. She had grown up in Germany for the first twelve years of her life before coming to the UK, and she'd struggled to make friends at school. She found people, feelings and emotions difficult to manage, and sometimes, when she was overwhelmed by feelings, would cut herself on her arms to help manage her emotions. She'd had, at least according to her father, who accompanied her to the appointment, a better experience at secondary school, once she learned the language. She played on the netball team, hung out with the other girls when she could and at weekends played football. She had two older sisters, to whom she was close.

Seda, though, saw things differently. She had not much liked secondary school either, and told me that she had increasingly felt like she was in the wrong body, that her female identity didn't sit comfortably with her. I tried to imagine what it might be like. I wondered how long I would manage if I had to dress in female clothes every day and present myself as a woman, despite feeling inside like a man. I think it would be hard to bear and quickly feel quite demoralising.

It became clear, as the consultation progressed, that there were three different agendas in the room: Seda's, mine and her family's.

Her family, represented by her father, could not make sense of her decision. She had always seemed such a happy girl, he said. In front of my eyes I could see him wilting, lamenting the loss of his daughter and the expectations he had of her life and his, perhaps thinking of the white bridal dress and grandchildren. He seemed simply baffled by the turn of events, and when he talked to her, he seemed to alternate between the name he had given her and the name she had chosen for herself.

Seda was by now starting work in landscape gardening and was dressed in a way such that her gender was not apparent. She had colourful tattoos on her arms, and scars on them too when you looked closely. We were separated by a generation, and perhaps a whole set of values, of my more conventional social conservatism and her more liberated indifference to convention. But her agenda was straightforward, which was for me to agree that she was unaffected by mental illness and should be able to proceed with her gender reassignment. She was entirely at ease with her decision, which had been accepted by her friends and which helped her make sense of her life.

For my own part, I was keen to do what I felt was the most responsible and professional thing, but I could see that almost whatever I did, someone was going to end up frustrated and perhaps resentful. I noted that her gender dysphoria was in the context of a particular personality type. She was someone who did not always understand her own emotional world and had never had a very strong sense of self. I felt that this might need exploring in more detail first, which was the decision I went with, and in so doing managed to upset both her and her father. Whilst not a brave decision, it was not obviously a wrong one either. Given the permanent nature of the course of action about to be taken, and given the potential contributory factors of mental health issues, I didn't see what else I could do. It was uncomfortable, but I had to acknowledge that sometimes underlying mental health issues can be lost or subsumed under a trans label. In some cases, autistic traits and personality variables influence an individual's sense of self, and this can include gender, although changing gender does not always resolve the inner turmoil. Without at least considering the issue of gender in the broader context of someone's life and personality, I would not necessarily be doing the right thing by the patient. When the power to make a significant decision that will affect someone's life for ever is in your hands professionally, asking difficult questions should not be seen as unkind or dismissive, although in the current climate one can be made to feel both of those things.

I have met other people who have struggled their whole lives, feeling that their gender was wrong, but who have never really wanted to explore surgery or live as the opposite gender. It has just created a sense of shame that they carry around within them, and which in some cases progresses from self-loathing to depression. What comes across most strongly in such consultations is the emotional pain they are in.

Most people I see with gender issues are not activists, not political, just deeply unhappy. Often they just wish that it had never happened to them this way, and they just want to be 'normal'. It is a world away from the noisy debates in the public arena.

Within psychiatry, there are some parallels between the issues around gender and those with the trajectory of homosexuality a generation ago. Gender identity disorders have until recently been classified under mental health disorders in the International Classification of Diseases (ICD-10). There has been at least one high-profile psychiatrist who has campaigned for gender identity disorders to remain as a psychiatric diagnosis, arguing that gender identity disorders are disorders of 'assumption'.[13] He compared the transgender self-identity to that of anorexia, in which the individual's self-perception has gone awry. This argument has not persuaded the medical profession, and the recently updated ICD-11 placed them under the category of 'gender incongruence' in the chapter 'Conditions related to sexual health' and removed them from the category of mental health disorders.[14]

The other similarity with homosexuality is the associated mental problems. Again, it is hard to know whether it is the same circular process causing psychiatric issues in trans communities as it was for homosexual communities. A group who are marginalised and often treated with a lack of consideration will understandably feel alienated from society. This can lead to isolation and shame, which are predisposing factors for mental health problems.

A number of psychiatric diagnoses are associated with a transgender population, including anxiety disorders, depression and psychosis,[15] and stigma seems to be associated with worse psychological outcomes.[16] One study showed higher rates of autism and neurodevelopmental disorders in the transgender population, as well as other psychiatric conditions.[17] What is cause and what is effect is not clear. Are increased rates of reported autism traits a consequence of societal rejection and alienation? Or is it that autistic people conform less to societal norms?[17] And are the increased mental health problems a consequence of internalised shame and feelings of societal rejection or, conversely, do mental health problems and alienation somehow lead to identification with being transgender?

There is some data suggesting that suicide rates may be higher in a transgender population. One large Danish study showed a rate of suicide attempts among transgender individuals 6.6 times that of the rest of the population, and a rate of suicide deaths almost three times higher.[18] However, another study found that when other mental health problems are accounted for, there is no longer an increased rate of suicide, and that gender dysphoria alone did not predict increased suicide risk.[19]

It is difficult to know where the transgender discussions will eventually settle in the public arena. But inevitably the current waves of anger and defiance on both sides of the debate will gradually subside, and there will be something of a realignment of the social contract, as there was for homosexuality.

I am not sure that the contribution of psychiatry has always been helpful to the debate over the years, although now at least the profession does seem to be trying to be fair to the evidence and considerate of the feelings of people struggling through life with the uncertainties and difficulties of who they are. We don't always have to endorse all the arguments of those with whom we disagree, but there are undoubtedly situations where a psychiatric assessment is important. We do, and should, have a legitimate interest in any area where psychiatric illness is increased, even if some of this itself is being driven by social pressures on people who are different. And I think we need to be able to offer a perspective when it is possible that a transgender identity may be a reflection of a more passing issue – a current state of distress or a need to rebel – for which more permanent treatments may be misguided. My hope is that disagreements can be respectful and, as far as possible, based on the evidence, but then I've always been an optimist.

11

Welcome to the Metaverse

When I saw Rina, it was at a virtual appointment towards the end of the COVID-19 pandemic lockdowns. At that stage, my appointments were nearly always online, but it still always felt a bit strange. Personal connection was often harder to make and, especially at the start, there were technical issues. The audio would begin to buffer at crucial moments. I would see someone's face crease up with tears as they spoke of a personal tragedy, then the image would freeze on the screen. Sometimes it would be as people began to tell me about suicidal thoughts. I would then have to wait, jaw clenched in frustration, until the system caught up. I would have to ask them to repeat what they had said and hope that the same thing didn't happen again.

In a different way though, virtual appointments would allow an insight into people's home life that you couldn't get at a face-to-face appointment in the hospital outpatient department. You could see inside their homes and the comings and goings. There was the appearance of pets, relatives, friends dropping by, all of which slowed the whole appointment down but did help to give a flavour to that intangible context of someone's life. On one occasion, a patient's mother wandered across the shot with a laundry basket, adding a correction to the patient's narrative as she headed to the washing machine.

Rina was in a busily decorated front room of her parents' house, on her own. She was nineteen and between school and university, having taken a gap year after completing school. Her plans to travel abroad to India, where her extended family lived, had been scuppered by the pandemic. She spent her time at home, like the rest of the country that year, now counting down the months until her university course started. She told me that she had begun to develop tics over the past six months. These were already evident within moments of the consultation starting. I could see her head jerking downwards, and there was repeated shrugging of the shoulders, blinking, throat clearing, whistling and swearing. As she began to tell me about them, her tics intensified.

Life had been difficult for her since the onset of her tics. She had stopped cooking because she would drop or throw the ingredients, such as bags of flour, across the room. On a night out, she had almost started a fight by swearing at strangers in a pub. At home, she had thrown a glass of water over her younger brother, apparently unable to suppress the impulse. Her narrative was delivered amidst a blizzard of eye blinking, head twitching and sudden obscenities. Sometimes, if the conversation was steered away from the tics and associated difficulties, they would settle down. Her parents were sympathetic but exasperated. Her friends and boyfriend were solidly supportive. They had accepted that she had some kind of disability and tried not to judge her.

It was hard not to sympathise with her. Strangely though, she seemed less concerned than I might have expected of someone with this burden of symptoms. She smiled as she recounted the events. Perhaps she was being stoical, but it was striking nevertheless. Her symptoms were rapidly becoming the central and defining feature of her life. As far as I could make out, hers was not a neurological illness but rather a psychological one. The tics did not fit with the typical Tourette's pattern. I could see from the electronic notes system that this was also the conclusion reached by the neurologist whom she had seen.

When it comes to tics and diseases like Tourette's syndrome, the diagnosis is largely a clinical one, which is to say that investigations don't really have much to add. It can be difficult, even for experienced doctors, to fully tell apart a diagnosis of neurologically caused tics from psychologically driven ones just by looking at the patient. One study showed that doctors watching videos of people with tics often did not agree about which were likely to be neurological and which were not.[1] They did better when they were given a little more information about the person with tics. There are differences, if you know what you are looking for.

I have seen people with tic disorders over many years, commonly with a diagnosis of Tourette's syndrome. The majority have been men (there is a four-to-one ratio of males to females), with tics beginning in childhood, mostly in the form of movements, such as twitching in the face, and other tics emerging over time. At first, parents can think their child is just being naughty or attention-seeking, before it gradually becomes apparent that the tics are involuntary. The tics can evolve in intensity to more complicated but pointless movements, like saluting or jumping. Sometimes, after the physical tics develop, verbal ones follow. These often start with grunting or throat clearing. They can go on to particular words and phrases coming out unexpectedly and inappropriately. The tics have the potential to cause social embarrassment, although people with Tourette's can usually suppress a tic for a short while at the expense of rising tension. The tic will then come out later, in an explosive kind of way, and quickly the inner tension eases. Tics normally improve as the child grows up, making it very unusual for Tourette's to start in late teenage or early adult years.

By contrast, psychologically driven tics tend to begin in the mid- to late teens and are far more common in girls and young women.[2] Their presentation is much more dramatic too. Patients with psychologically driven tics do not seem to be able to suppress them in the way that those with Tourette's can.[2,3] This was what led to Rina throwing food around the kitchen when trying to cook a simple meal. There was also her repetitive swearing. This symptom is often associated with Tourette's but is actually not as common as usually supposed. Studies put impulsive swearing in Tourette's at around 15–20% of patients. Obscene gestures, such as giving someone the middle finger, are even lower at around 5%.[2] Compare this to the rate of swearing or obscene gestures in psychologically driven tics, which was as high as 93% in one study. The same study found that psychological tics were much more severe and disabling than those normally seen in Tourette's (and, slightly bizarrely, over half of those in the study had the same vocal tic of saying the word 'beans'[3]).

The diagnosis given to presentations like Rina's, at least informally, was TikTok tics. These were part of a rapid expansion of such presentations that had spiked over the COVID-19 pandemic. There were several academic papers that almost simultaneously published similar findings. Once I started to look into it, the figures were quite shocking. There was clearly a kind of social contagion happening. Apparently, a number of social influencers with symptoms of Tourette's syndrome were appearing on TikTok and other platforms. They were often florid and dramatic, and not like any presentation of Tourette's syndrome that I had seen. These were not niche videos either. One study reported, 'Within a 3-week period in March of 2021, views of videos with the keywords #tourette and #tic increased by 7% to a total of 5.8 billion views.'[3] That is an extraordinary number. It would only take a tiny percentage of vulnerable, impressionable or anxious people to watch these videos and start to be affected by them to create the kind of wave we were seeing. Another study reported that sudden-onset tic disorders in teenage girls referred to one specialist clinic in London had increased from about four to six per year to three to four per week.[4] A similar phenomenon was observed in North America and other European countries.

Medicine and the course of disease are constantly changed by our different cultural and social environments. Industrial lung diseases such as asbestosis or silicosis are associated with the industrial revolution. Smoking-related diseases have soared over the last century. The current obesity crisis in the Western world is accelerating many of the related diseases such as diabetes, heart disease, stroke and osteoarthritis. In the 1980s, when I was growing up, repetitive strain injuries were the new health crisis.[5] These resulted from overuse of specific parts of the body, for example, in the hands and arms caused by typing. There was even a wrist injury that became known as 'Rubik's wrist', caused by the overuse of the Rubik's Cube. Later, the use of new and synthesised drugs such as ketamine created new medical problems, for example, 'ketamine bladder'. There are countless examples. Progress in society changes the landscape of disease. Old diseases become rare or are eliminated, such as cholera or typhoid, only to be replaced by new ones. Tell me what your diseases are, and I'll tell you what decade you're living in.

The effect that societal progress has on our minds is harder to define. It lacks the clear narrative of diseases such as silicosis. Yet one recurring question is whether the internet, one of the most significant social changes of recent decades, is the cause of escalating levels of mental illness. The topic is the subject of agonised debate in the media. Is our dependence on the internet, in all its guises, our excessive use of it, fuelling the current mental health crisis?

It is all but impossible to function in the modern world without accessing at least some aspect of cyberspace. The inability to do so is to risk exclusion in the workplace and to make nearly impossible the myriad of day-to-day activities such as paying bills, shopping and communications. My father, until his recent stroke still driving, would rage against parking apps. He was the only man I knew who carried a little transparent bag of change in his glove compartment for the parking meter. The gradual phasing out of parking meters in favour of online parking and apps made him dread driving anywhere that there was paid parking. Lacking internet access or technological know-how is an impediment to being able to engage in society. For most households, reliable internet is a utility like water and energy.

I am one of the digital immigrants, people who grew up in a pre-internet world. I remember having to learn what the internet was. I had to attend a series of training courses at work to be taught how to use a computer, create Word documents and spreadsheets, and send an email. Nothing was intuitive. The legacy of my late introduction to the cyberworld is evident in my two-fingered pecking on the computer keyboard, which both amuses and frustrates my children. The sound of it carries into the next room. My interaction with the computer is a bit like someone who has learned to speak another language. I'm pretty fluent, broadly competent, but never quite able to shake off the accent that places me as an outsider.

The current generation, who have never lived in a world without the internet, are digital natives. They have been exposed to influences that previous generations would have taken decades to see, if at all. Social media provides platforms for all types of views. In my generation, we had the pub bore. They sat in the same place, ordered the same drink and had a narrow range of views both poorly thought out and loudly expressed. They would buttonhole reluctant patrons with their views on whatever topic they were currently expert in. The pub bore would have been humoured, perhaps with eyes casting desperately around to find a sociably acceptable means of escape.

Now, the pub bore, the closet racist, the misinformed, the wilfully destructive and the prejudiced all have a variety of platforms to connect with like-minded individuals and influence (and often poison) the public debate. Yet the problems go beyond the coarsening of public debate. There are the conspiracy theorists, the sellers of snake oils, the unscrupulous grifters and the influencers. There are the malevolent, the gullible and the desperate. Health information can be put out by anyone, to say more or less whatever they like, with no quality control whatsoever or consequences. It ranges from the absurd to the misleading, to the actively harmful. It is a battle that many in the medical profession do not realise is being fought, let alone being lost.

I first came across the darker underside of the internet in the late 1990s, before most people had even heard of Google. I was in a small classroom lecture about eating disorders. As part of the talk, the specialist in eating disorders showed us slides of web pages from anorexia websites, which were a new phenomenon to most of us. These 'pro-ana' sites existed to promote anorexia. It was shocking and it was upsetting. They seemed to celebrate a serious disorder and, even worse, encourage others to follow down that path. Typically, these sites contained a 'tips and tricks' section, giving advice on weight loss, such as fasting or use of diet pills. Advice on purging was offered, including laxative abuse or how to make yourself sick. Tips were given to avoid hunger (people with anorexia, contrary to what is sometimes believed, are ravenous), like drinking water to feel temporarily full. People shared methods for finding effective ways of lying or concealing symptoms and behaviours from others who may be concerned.[6,7]

Another feature of the pro-ana websites was the 'thinspiration' galleries. These were defined in one study as 'inspirational photo galleries and quotes that aim to serve as motivators for weight loss'.[7] The images we saw in the lecture were of young women skeletally thin, skin and bones, emaciated like the photos of concentration camp survivors, or the cachectic end-stage cancer patients I saw on the wards. Even then, I was a pretty battle-hardened doctor, but it was one of the few times I've had to turn away from what I was watching. It was just too upsetting.

Perhaps most galling of all was the complete lack of accountability for the websites. These sites unashamedly promoted a fearsome disease with pretty well the highest mortality rate of any psychiatric illness.[8] The messages that pro-ana websites (and, later, 'pro-mia' websites promoting bulimia) put into the world could not have been propagated without the internet, because in any other regulated medium, such harmful information would have been rapidly shut down.

We have known for some time that social contagion is a significant influence in the development of anorexia. This traditionally has been through teen or fashion magazines celebrating thinness as an ideal in women, albeit they were not explicitly promoting anorexia but a lifestyle in which looks and low weight were associated with beauty. As the ways in which people interacted with media evolved, from print and television to the internet and social media, the ways in which harm could accrue escalated.

The effects of the pro-ana websites were predictable. In one study, undergraduates were shown pro-ana websites. The students exposed to these websites reported lower mood and self-esteem, and they perceived themselves as heavier compared with people who did not see them.[9] A separate study explored their effects on the calorie intake of healthy female students. Some students were shown the pro-ana websites, some were shown healthy exercise websites and others were shown a neutral website for tourists.

Worryingly, after seeing the pro-ana websites, students significantly reduced their calorie intake, with a marked difference in the overall calories consumed compared with before. Even with this glancing exposure to pro-ana sites, the effect persisted for three weeks beyond the end of the study.[10]

Female teenagers appear to be the most vulnerable to this kind of content.[11] The increase of anorexia in this group over recent decades is likely to be explained, at least in part, by social media. This includes not only the pro-ana websites, but pressures from the inescapable rise of models and influencers, and photographic filters that distort and flatter, all of which lead to unattainable standards that teenagers feel a pressure to meet. They are at an age when fitting in and being accepted is especially important, and self-esteem is bound up with peer group acceptance and looks. Either way, there is no doubting the effects of social media on the real-world behaviours of individuals, and as always, it is the most insecure and vulnerable who are at the highest risk.

Our journey into the virtual world has only increased over time. The arrival of COVID-19 accelerated the change. Living online affected people in different ways. For my own part, during the pandemic I began to think of virtual meetings as a kind of death. Any connection I had with others was made in the ethereal world, where minds met but there was no physical substance. Badly lit, spectral figures would loom into view on my screen. Poor-quality, glitchy audio would accompany the images. I began to feel strangely upset by the disconnection from reality. Yet my own existential unease did not come close to the more profound loss of social connections that children were experiencing. Many papers highlighted the rise of depression in particular and also anxiety disorders in under-eighteens.[12, 13] For children of school age, the pandemic lockdowns were having a profound impact. They were affecting their education undoubtedly, but also their socialisation at a time in their lives when their friendship groups were their world. Their virtual world was their only world, and this was a place into which many fell in deep.

TikTok tics were one of the most widespread and unusual effects of this sudden dependence on the virtual world and, if not a frequent referral to my clinics, became a regular one over the following couple of years. Rina believed that her diagnosis was Tourette's syndrome. In fact, that was one of the first things she said to me in the consultation. Sometimes Tourette's can exist alongside the new, psychological type of tics. In Rina's case though, I didn't feel there was much room for doubt. As I explained to her, psychologically driven symptoms are not the same as making them up. The mind and brain are too closely connected and the interactions too nuanced to make some 'real' versus 'fake' distinctions. There was no evidence that Rina was deliberately putting any of this on. She did not appear to be fully in control of what she was doing. She believed that she had developed an illness that may be lifelong, and my suggestions that this may not have an organic, physical cause were met with polite scepticism. I was to an extent sympathetic with her position. It is not intuitive to think that a very physical presentation has no underlying bodily cause.

The more formal diagnosis for Rina was a 'functional disorder'. This is a relatively new term, given to people who present with physical, often neurological-looking symptoms, but where no physical cause is found. Examination of patients will usually reveal some inconsistencies between the deficits that the patient complains of and the findings on physical examination. There will sometimes be evidence too of psychological factors that are driving the symptoms. Neurologists often explain this to patients using the analogy of a computer. In this case, the brain and spinal cord, and so forth, are the 'hardware'. They are the wires and the expensive kit. Functional neurological disorders, neurologists explain, are not a hardware problem. There's nothing identifiably wrong with the nerves, no missing bits on the MRI of the head, and all the hardware appears to be intact. Functional disorders are rather something to do with the software.

Although the analogy sounds good, it is not always clear what we mean by 'software'. For computers, software is lines of code. In human function, it is much harder to articulate. In people, it is something about mind, volition, subconscious processes, learned behaviour. Childhood experience of illness and its perceived seriousness and cause can be important factors. Mood and anxiety will both influence the performance of the human software. There is something too about how the brain predicts what will happen and, in this, the predictions can become self-serving and maintain symptoms, like tics, even in the absence of disease. Human software is thus far more ephemeral, intangible and imprecise than written code. Yet for all its imprecision, nobody doubts the influence of the mind, the human software, on the development of symptoms.

Functional disorders are the successors of the diagnoses that have previously been called 'hysterical' or 'conversion disorders'. These describe symptoms that appear to be physical, often neurological, but examination and investigation find no evidence of a physical cause. These can include paralysis, seizures, numbness, floaters in the visual field, loss of voice, amongst a variety of others. Both terms, hysteria and conversion disorder, reflected the time in which they were described. The diagnosis of hysteria, which supposed that the wanderings of the uterus caused the various neurological symptoms, was a legacy from antiquity. The theory was a less satisfactory explanation for the men who got this disorder. This difficulty was largely resolved by pretending that they didn't. And so, the name persisted over many centuries until the illness was redefined by the psychoanalysts in the twentieth century.

Psychoanalysts like Freud understood the disorder as the consequence of some internalised conflict. This repressed conflict would be 'converted' into a physical symptom, sometimes with a symbolic representation of the conflict itself. Loss of voice may follow after having said something hateful or unforgivable, for example. This has given way to our current understanding. Functional neurological disorders are far more nuanced. They describe the complex interaction of physical and psychological states, the 'hardware' and 'software', which both need to work for the individual to function normally. And as a side note, it's interesting to me that analogies for illness, or the way they are understood, are always in relation to the latest technology. Currently it's computers, but in the past it was pulleys, hydraulics, or electricity, and in the future we will no doubt make analogies with quantum mechanics.

For all the concern about TikTok tics, social contagion is hardly new and it doesn't need the internet to help it spread. Ideas, beliefs and behaviours can be spread by social contact, proclamations or religious authority. There are countless examples of epidemics of illness arising over the centuries. In the late medieval period, dancing plagues intermittently sprung up in Europe. Although sounding faintly comical, these were not benign events. They were driven by a deep supernatural fear of punishment, and those affected would dance themselves into a state of exhaustion over days on end. A *Lancet* paper exploring these dancing plagues found that certain conditions were met whenever dance contagion took place.[14] The first was a belief in the concept of a dancing curse, that it was real and could affect them. The second was a state of emotional or physical distress that made people suggestible. After that, all it took was a spark to ignite the 'dancing, leaping, and hopping', for example, a belief that people indeed had been cursed.

In this respect, there are parallels with the TikTok tics. Each new technology brings its own mechanism of spreading ideas that

somehow filter into the consciousness of individuals in a population, who may then develop beliefs that they claim to have arisen
independently, without realising the myriad influences from the
world around them by which they were led to them. In the case
of the TikTok tics, it started with exposure to tics and a belief
that they were common. It is relevant that the people promoting
or instantiating the tics were social media influencers, for many
young people the priests of our time. Secondly, the conditions of
the COVID-19 pandemic provided a unique period of psychological vulnerability. Within this context, it would not take much
for the symptoms to begin. They may start, perhaps, by indulging
in an inner urge to move, shout out or twitch. After that, a belief
that the person has been affected by tics can start to take hold. An
internal focus on the need to move or vocalise can exacerbate the
problem, and after a while, the symptoms just run on their own,
involuntarily and without even thinking about it.

New technologies always cause a moral panic. But the number
of uses we have for the internet and the fact that it is accessible
to nearly everyone all of the time have opened up something of
a Pandora's box of possible harms. And, inevitably, these tend to
be given plausible-sounding diagnostic labels, which quickly gain
popular currency precisely because of the internet. One of the most
recent concerns has been about 'internet gaming disorder'. Over
the years, stories have appeared in the press concerning teenagers
and young men playing games compulsively. One story reported
a man having died after a three-day online gaming binge.[15] It was
the second reported death that year in Taiwan attributed to online
gaming. A study set out to find the number of deaths attributed
to internet gaming, and found twenty-three cases between 2002
and 2021.[16] These were thought to relate to a variety of factors
including sitting for long periods of time, dehydration, changes in
blood pressure because of the games, and exhaustion. Each death

was an individual tragedy, but taken together they did not constitute an epidemic.

There is mixed evidence concerning the addictiveness of internet games. Despite the exponential increase in internet exposure in recent years, as well as the increased sophistication of internet games, the development of problematic online gaming has not changed much between 1998 and 2016.[17] This, as the authors of the study comment, is unlike addictions such as gambling, for which as the opportunity to engage increases (for example, more betting shops or online casinos in the case of gambling), the rate of addiction also tends to increase.

A study published in the *American Journal of Psychiatry* sounded a similarly cautious note. Some 160 million Americans play internet games. If current criteria to diagnose internet gaming disorder were used, the researchers estimated this would result in up to one million Americans who would now need help. Yet there was no strong evidence that those who met the criteria for gaming addiction were particularly disadvantaged in terms of their emotional outcomes. And defining it as a disorder in this way would have practical implications. Any funding for the treatment of internet gaming disorder would need to compete for the limited pot of money allocated to serious mental illness.[18]

My own experience of video gaming was in the lonely days of being a junior doctor. I worked unsociable hours, and I am not sure I would have used the games to socialise anyway. I just needed a way of emptying my head of all the brutal reality I was exposed to day after day. The sheer volume, the pain, the fear, the misery of patients coming to casualty or admitted to hospital was overwhelming. I found retreat in my Nintendo 64. I started to think about it all day long, to the extent that when I saw CCTV cameras mounted high up in the hospital car park, the only thing that I thought about was getting the sniper rifle from my James

Bond game inventory and taking them out. I almost lived the game. After around two years of intensive playing, it was something almost banal that made me stop. On the start-up for a game called Banjo-Kazooie, whilst the game was loading, there would appear on the screen a counter showing the cumulative hours that the game had been played. I used to frantically tap 'A' on my controller to quickly go past that screen. One day, though, the game got stuck there, and I could see how many hundreds of hours I'd spent playing. All the days, weeks even, of my life I would never get back, lost in a trivial pursuit, the voluntary removal of myself from the world. That was the moment I felt I couldn't keep on playing. It is hard now to relate to that urge to play. I have neither the time nor interest to invest in a vast make-believe world. The prospect of learning the various buttons, triggers and bumpers on the controllers makes my shoulder sag when my children challenge me. For some at least, what might appear to be an unhealthy use of video games is something that they naturally grow out of.

It is not always easy to differentiate those people who play internet games intensively because they enjoy them from those who play because they have a problem. Despite the panic about the loss of socialisation with peers during the COVID-19 pandemic, for many children and adolescents internet gaming is the very thing that keeps them connected with their peers, and I would consider that healthy. Perhaps the key component of whether someone has a problem is when playing is causing significant detriment to their life. Even then, you'd need to be sure it wasn't because of another mental illness, such as depression, that internet gaming is masking. There has been trenchant opposition to the inclusion of internet gaming disorder in the diagnostic lexicon. In one widely cited paper in the *Journal of Behavioural Addictions*,[19] the authors argued that it risked drawing children and adolescents into being diagnosed with a mental health disorder. It also risked becoming a fixed entity, so that future research would focus on confirming the extent of the problem, rather than the validity of the diagnosis. Finally, the authors considered the waste of public resources with the potential over-inclusiveness of the diagnosis. As one psychiatrist was quoted as saying, 'I don't think it's in anyone's interest to label a 13-year-old who's screaming, wanting to play *Minecraft* as an "addict".'[20]

These dilemmas are why, in the end, the American classification DSM decided against including internet gaming as a mental health diagnosis, although the ICD did decide to include it as a 'gaming disorder'. In the UK, there are now clinics to treat it. Despite the potentially large numbers who may fit its criteria, only a very small minority are likely to need treatment. Which of course leads to the question, why would the definition of the disorder need to be so broad if the number needing treatment is so limited?

Psychiatry has not found a way to think about behavioural addictions and whether they should truly be considered as addictions. I think most psychiatrists would recognise gambling addictions as something more clearly psychiatric, in many ways closer to substance abuse than anything else. The cognitive testing, brain imaging and heritability are similar to those for substance addictions.[21] Yet there are many other more modern 'addictions' that may be best thought of as part of life, otherwise the whole edifice of addictions would collapse under the weight of behaviours that most people would think of as normal. Sex addiction is one example. There is little evidence to support this as an addiction. DSM-5 did not include sex addiction at all in the most recent psychiatric classification, and as we have seen, DSM generally errs on over-inclusion rather than under-inclusion. In the rival ICD-11, sex addiction was included under 'impulse control disorders', described as 'repeated failure to resist an impulse, drive, or urge to perform an act that is rewarding to the person'.[22]

This leads to something of a philosophical question. What are our responsibilities to control our own impulses? And to what extent should our inability to do so be considered a mental disorder, as opposed to a reflection of our own decisions, which we could control if we chose to and indeed did in the past? This is exactly the problem with expanding diagnostic boundaries. Although the intention is commonly noble, to allow people to get help for problems that they would otherwise not have done, it can lead to people dissociating themselves from the consequences of their actions because they are 'ill'. That is not to say that they can't cause an individual difficulties in their life, but so can a lot of things that aren't mental health problems, like consistently spending money unwisely, poor choice of relationships or driving too fast.

When it comes to concerns about behavioural addictions, smartphone addiction has steadily climbed the rankings. Parents' forums are full of anxiety about how to control or even monitor smartphone use. At work, I have noticed with medical students that during any lull in a conversation or teaching, there is almost a reflex for them to reach for their phones. In fact, I have noticed myself doing it now. When I wake in the night, I check emails, newspaper websites, social media. If asked, I would probably say that I am addicted to my mobile phone, and I think many others would say the same about themselves.

Much has been written about smartphone addiction in the academic literature. Rating scales have been created and tested,[23] and population surveys have set out the scale of the problem. When I tested myself on one of the scales, unsurprisingly I fell on the wrong side of the addiction border ('Using my smartphone longer than I had intended?'; 'Feeling impatient and fretful when I am not holding my smartphone?' Both definitely yes, and so on), which would put me in the category of smartphone addiction. In this, I am in good company, with 39% of young adults in one UK study also appearing to be suffering from smartphone addiction.[24]

Another study, this time looking at the global picture, recorded highest levels of smartphone addiction in China and Saudi Arabia (around 35%) and lowest in France and Germany (around 20%). The UK was somewhere in the middle.[25] The question though is how helpful the diagnosis of smartphone addiction is. What is it really telling us? To my way of thinking, it says that there is a new and very helpful technology that also doubles up as entertainment. There is a range of use, from infrequent to very frequent, and there are a variety of reasons why this is so. Personally, I get bored quickly, and a smartphone is the perfect way to be constantly entertained. I would also rather do almost anything than go to bed. Yes, there are days when I would have got more sleep without having a mobile phone, particularly when I wake up in the night and decide to check on X/Twitter or play Wordle. Yet I do a lot of work via my mobile, learn another language via Duolingo and use it instead of television.

Concern about smartphone addiction brings into focus the usefulness and validity of the term, and what it represents. It runs the risk, as do many such panics, of creating a new term and then believing that it represents something real and troublesome. Such diagnoses tend to develop their own gravitational pull, so that more research about smartphone addiction is funded, more papers written, more findings disseminated, and a reality is now established. One paper argued, 'A behavior may have a similar presentation as addiction . . . but that does not mean that it should be considered an addiction.'[26] Herein lies the problem. I think we have got to the stage where we are too quick to label behaviours as addictive and embark down a pathway of illness and treatment, rather than consider the wider social issues. Excessive smartphone use may occasionally cause problems, but if over 30% of the population have 'problematic use', then something doesn't add up.

Moral panics are constantly evolving, and at the time each seems warranted, dressed in the social concerns of the day. When I was growing up, people were quick to blame television for the drop in social standards. This current one, of zombified youth staring at a screen, is increasingly being spoken of as an explanation for current mental health problems. But we have not established the direction of causality – are troubled people using smartphones more, or does smartphone use really cause mental illness?

The internet has given rise to a number of other new, catchy-sounding diagnoses. Snapchat dysmorphia is a term given to people wanting to look like their digitally manipulated (filtered) images on sites like Instagram and Snapchat. Muscle dysmorphia, or 'bigorexia', is another proposed diagnosis. It is a condition in which men think they are too skinny, not 'manly' enough. Excessive workouts, dieting and preoccupation with physique are typical behaviours,[27] which follow a social trend that idealises muscular men. Even male action toys have become more muscular over the past thirty years.[28] This mirrors social changes, as the idealised male shape has become more worked out, with bigger chests and increased muscle mass. Predictably, dire warnings of the extent of the problem have followed. Estimates of the incidence of muscle dysmorphia in US military personnel were 12.7% for men and 4.2% for women.[27]

The list goes on. 'Orthorexia' is the current obsession for healthy eating. One study found a prevalence rate of 6.9% in the population.[29] Orthorexia is driven by our cultural climate and abetted by social media. Influencers promote their dietary stringencies under the superficially appealing notion of clean living, yet the drive for perfect health only becomes unhealthier as the food choices become more extreme. It seems a peculiarly modern affliction. It is resonant of a society that has lost its way, the previous cares of life, income, security and shelter now taken for granted. Yet instead of enjoying a level of prosperity unimaginable to previous generations, there is a need in many to find something else to fight against. It's the sort of Californian mindset that makes billionaires squander their wealth on an elixir that will make them live for ever.

Wanting to be healthy is entirely sensible and understandable. A preoccupation with only healthy foods is not. It becomes unscientific and antisocial. As people become more obsessional about their food choices, it leads to them becoming more isolated. As the authors of one paper put it: 'The causes of orthorexia, which are often hidden behind a very deep and seemingly attractive belief, may be found in the illusion of total health, with no pathological risks, the desire for total control of one's own life.'[29]

When I think of the diagnoses that have followed our move into the metaverse, I am reminded of those old screen savers. Those were the fractal patterns that appear to come towards the screen, and as they arrive, they begin again as a dot in the distance. There is an illusion of change, but fundamentally things are the same. Every generation faces its unique challenges, and the social environment will shape the behaviour of individuals within it. To those vulnerable, the behaviours can become extreme. TikTok tics, orthorexia, bigorexia, internet gaming may not be the diseases themselves but just the outward symptoms of an underlying problem that would have existed in any generation. In some, they are passing phases, just as dressing as a punk, mod or goth would have been. There is a danger in rushing to pathologise them. One research group in Oxford, considering the question of whether the widespread adoption of internet technologies has fuelled a rise in mental health problems, did not find any consistent changes in either well-being or mental health over a twenty-year period.[30]

The study seemed to go against the grain of the current narrative, that everything is getting worse and we are losing a generation to the perils of modern life. We worry that we may have created an environment for our youth of war, violence, peril, lack of education, lack of opportunity, and danger. The fears of cyberspace and technological advances, of addictions and poor attention span, are part of the current anxieties. We need to treat those who need help, but equally, we need to be very wary about labelling whole swathes of the population as having a mental illness or addiction.

12

Risk

Being a psychiatrist involves looking after people at moments of crisis in their life, often when they are mentally at their lowest or most distressed. In the peak of their mental anguish, staring into the fog of an uncertain future, people often tell me that they don't know if they want to carry on living. It is important not to overreact in those moments. People need to be able to talk to someone who is really listening, someone who is not going to immediately fall into risk management mode. Managing risk takes time, patience and a level of trust, for the patient to be able to open up to the doctor, but also the other way round. As a doctor, you need to have confidence that the patient is telling you the truth, and not holding back what is really going on for them. Missteps here can have far-reaching consequences. Yet risk assessments have become, to my mind, a barometer of the state of mental health care. They are commonly routine, done quickly as a checklist of questions and reduce complexity into something overly simplistic. Is this high, medium or low risk? Yet ascribing a label and focusing on risk can take attention away from understanding the deeper underlying issues that matter to the individual. Done this way, risk assessments are liable to misrepresent the actual risk and alienate patients.

I remember seeing Camilla in my outpatient clinic one icy February morning. As I exited the hospital building in the direction of the nearby outpatient department where Camilla was waiting to see me, I was running a little late, which made me impatient (I have a thing about timekeeping). I tried to shuffle around a woman in front of me, who was walking very slowly and unevenly in the exact centre of the narrow path leading to the outpatient department. I felt strangely cross with her for delaying me, and as I finally got past her and sped up, I slipped on a thin sheet of ice and my feet went from under me, and I landed heavily on my back. The tower of notes I was carrying flew across the path onto the road, the batteries of my Dictaphone rolled to the edge of the pavement, and I lay there winded. The woman I had passed caught up with me, all concern and kindness. I felt ashamed of my uncharitable thoughts about her only moments before as she gathered up my notes, picked up the batteries from the slush and debris on the pavement, and helped me to my feet. As I trudged slowly to the outpatient department, the back of my suit was wet through, my trousers were sticking to me and my tie was splashed with mud.

Whether it was this inauspicious prelude or something else that made me remember the appointment so clearly I couldn't say, but the case has stuck in my mind. I doubt I would have remembered the same case in subsequent years, when the scenario Camilla described had become so normalised. She was already in the waiting room, a woman in her late thirties, and looked up as I walked in. As she was the only person waiting, she followed me to the upstairs consulting room, with wooden panels, an old-fashioned wooden desk with an ink blotter, and a nautical-looking clock above the door. It felt like we were having a consultation in the captain's quarters of an ancient schooner.

Camilla sat down on the chair in front of the desk and took in the room. I put my notes on the desk, walked round to my side, pulled my chair up and then gasped as I banged my knee on the desk drawer, which was positioned uncomfortably low. I had lost count of the number of times I'd done that. Camilla smiled, and after some small talk about the icy weather, we got on with the consultation. She began by recalling her breast cancer diagnosis a few years previously. She hadn't been married long and had been desperate to start a family, so when the diagnosis was made one spring afternoon almost four years before our appointment, the bottom fell out of her world. She told me the story of her cancer diagnosis, a story she had told many times before, so that it came out coherently and with little emotion, at least at first. I jotted down notes as she talked. Many of the cancer diagnoses I hear about start in the same way. There is the moment of noticing a symptom, a niggling pain or lump that won't seem to clear up, accompanied by a sinking feeling counterbalanced by optimism that it's probably nothing, followed by the diagnosis and life being upended instantly. All the supposedly important things cease to be so, and waves of emotion hardly have time to find expression in the chaos before the patient submits themselves to the hospital system.

There is comfort in the hospital routine. The intense interest from the doctors, the planning, the cautious optimism, all provide a focus and distraction from the maelstrom of emotions. They bring the patient back into the present, guiding them through the flurry of activity. So it was with Camilla as she began her treatment – the endless round of blood tests, investigations, hospital admissions, surgery, daycare, chemotherapy. Her life was barely her own any more, and she bore it all with stoicism.

After one hospital admission to address some unexpected side effects of her medications, she came home to her husband, who sat her down and told her that he was leaving her. I looked up from my notes at her. More than the cancer, more than the treatment, she said, this was the thing that had hurt her the most. She clearly didn't want to cry, so she kept stopping her narrative, jaw tightening against the trembling that prefaces tears, until she felt ready to continue. She was haunted by the callous way her husband had spoken to her. One phrase in particular stuck in her mind, when her husband told her, 'This wasn't part of the deal.' It was hard to hear. At the very time when she needed the most support, it was taken away by the person she had most expected to rely on. As a psychiatrist, sympathetic neutrality is usually best when listening to a patient's narrative, but I felt indignant on her behalf. I resisted the urge to say that her husband quite literally *had* agreed to this deal;'in sickness and in health' had been part of his marriage vows, taken only a few years before.

Now nearing the end of treatment, Camilla felt bereft. Through the tough grind of the preceding months, she had kept her focus on the end of treatment, the promise of a new life with new priorities, the holiday she and her husband would go on, the family they would finally be able to start. The conversation paused. She picked up her handbag, which had been on the chair next to her, and put it on her knee. It looked like a shield, the tall leather bag covering half of her body. I imagined what she must have been thinking. Her expectations of life had been turned upside down, and her faith in men, humanity perhaps, shattered.

She told me that at that moment she could no longer see the point of carrying on. I wondered what the surgeons and oncologists would have made of this. The army of consultants, theatre staff, nurses, physiotherapists, junior doctors, ward nurses, administrators and many others who had worked as one to save the life of a woman who no longer wanted to be saved. All the meetings, the planning, the appointments, the operations, the investment in the future of a patient now on the brink of emotional collapse. Their job had been to focus on how she could live, rather than why. She described how she'd had an ample supply of medications from the hospital, including tablets for her cancer, painkillers and sleeping pills, which she had emptied out into her hand. Even as she held them, she didn't think she would do anything, but then there was a call from her husband ('He didn't even ask how I was.') to discuss some practicalities of their separation.

After the overdose, she woke up in the emergency department. She felt exhausted, sick and deeply ashamed. 'I didn't really want to die,' she told me. 'I was just so angry with him.' I nodded. It wasn't hard to understand, although I suspected that anger was a surface emotion, beneath which were the roiling waves of sadness, fear of the future, and despair.

After she was discharged from the hospital, she was visited by the Home Treatment Team, part of her local community mental health services. 'Always a different person every time,' she told me, 'and all they wanted to know was whether I was going to try and kill myself again.' Camilla wanted to talk, to help make sense of her life and find a way to move on, but instead of any meaningful engagement with her mental and emotional state, the appointments were focused on assessing whether she was at risk of suicide. As far as the mental health services were concerned, as long as there was no imminent risk, they'd done their job.

Camilla's experience is now commonplace, as interactions with patients have become shaped by a risk agenda, whereby hospitals and medical staff have been conditioned to prioritise the avoidance of adverse events like suicide as the primary goal of a consultation. So long as the patient cleared the bar and lived for a while longer, that would be good enough. There was no emphasis on the patient and their life, what made them unique, what talents they had and what aspirations they would like to develop. It was entirely negative, almost the inverse of care. And all of this was driven by a cultural agenda that risk was unacceptable and must always be managed and reduced. It meant that mental health professionals were starting to practise a kind of formulaic tick-box approach that served the systems and the statisticians but rarely the patient. The risk forms would be filled in, some comments would be recorded in the electronic notes, and it would be considered a successful patient encounter.

Many patients I speak to now feel that they're being treated like risky cost pressures to be managed, rather than living human beings with complex and often messy lives and relationships. This was what had brought Camilla to my clinic. She had no objection to seeing the community mental health team, but she had come to see me as a private patient because she didn't want to keep talking about a risk that was no longer there, and one that only reminded her of the misery and shame that she associated with the whole affair. She wanted to talk about now, the future and what mattered to her, rather than answer questions to satisfy the hospital system and its insurers.

It is hard for trainee psychiatrists now to imagine psychiatry without mandatory risk assessments. But they were not part of my training, at least not at first. I remember the first time a risk assessment form was introduced in my hospital, back in 1998, to a large meeting of bewildered psychiatrists. It was offered as a self-evident good, so there was no room for debate, and the forms were soon mandatory. Over the years the psychiatric preoccupation with risk has mushroomed. It now includes not only an individual's risk of harming themselves or others, but also their risk of radicalisation, terrorism, posing a threat to children, being subject to exploitation, and others. Lengthening mandatory forms require all these risks to be addressed for each patient.

Leaving aside whether psychiatrists can spot radicalisation, and what to do if we did think somebody was, for example, getting more religiously observant, where is the evidence that our risk assessments are accurate? The bad news is that pretty well every study examining this area shows that formulaic risk assessment forms are unhelpful and potentially misleading. Take suicide risk assessments. Meta-analyses show that risk assessment tools of the types that have commonly been used in the emergency department do not predict who will go on to die by suicide.[1] In fact, about half of suicides occur in individuals considered to be at low risk.[2] Conversely, of the patients considered at high risk when assessed, the vast majority will never attempt suicide.[2] You might think that these results, consistently produced by researchers over the years, would have discouraged the use of risk assessment scores, but you would be wrong. Time-consuming and unhelpful risk assessment forms must now be filled out. One study from my own hospital showed that suicide and violence risk assessments did not correlate with future risk,[3] and interestingly, the only thing that did predict the risk of future death in this study was self-neglect, something very rarely emphasised in risk assessments because it is the noisier, more florid psychoses or depression that attract the attention. The quieter, burnt-out individual with psychosis is unlikely to score high marks on a checklist of risk.

Unfortunately, the idea of risk has now become welded into the system. On a number of occasions, in my role as a trainer of junior psychiatrists, I have supervised a competent trainee's assessment of a patient, observed their careful delineation of the problem and formulation of a management plan. Then, as the patient interview draws to a close, there comes the panicky and jarring question, entirely out of context with the mood and tenor of the consultation, about whether they have ever considered suicide. I don't blame the junior psychiatrists, because they are only doing what they have been told, and their question is often asked with a tinge of anticipatory regret and apology, but the effect is hardly therapeutic. Patients who have never before engaged with psychiatry look a little startled and discomfited, worried that the wrong answer may get them taken into involuntary care. Patients who have been through the system before will often interrupt as the clunky introduction to the question gets under way, and say, 'No, I'm not going to kill myself,' thereby cutting the conversation short and leaving the doctor nodding awkwardly.

Camilla and I met half a dozen times over the next six months. She wondered if she had become mentally ill. I could understand her concern. Broadly, if you think of anxiety as a response to threat events and depression as a response to loss events, then Camilla had plenty of risk factors for mental illness. The threat of the cancer and everything this meant to her life and work would have predisposed her to an anxiety disorder, and the end of her relationship had brought her low. Yet aside from that brief moment of self-harm, her reactions were broadly within the normal range of human emotions. Her confidence, though, was shattered, and her expectations for her future life had been turned upside down. When real tragedy touches and brushes past someone, it is a rare person who remains unchanged. The trick is to turn this into a meaningful and productive change, rather than a retreat and withdrawal from the world.

Camilla did eventually start to adjust to her new reality. She learned how to cope with the waves of anxiety that accompanied hospital appointments and scans, and decided on an entirely new employment based on her love of literature. As to relationships, she warily dipped her toe into the water, but by the time I discharged her, she wasn't yet ready to dive in. What I had given her, in all honesty, was not that difficult to deliver. Mostly it was support, a sounding board and the reassurance that she was neither mentally ill nor permanently defined and tainted by what had happened. We explored issues of loss, betrayal and guilt; tried to understand how her husband had reacted; and considered what she wanted from her future. Yet it was a route that could only be navigated once the conversations about risk had been put to one side.

There is another aspect to these risk forms. They are driven by a desire to standardise. The UK workforce crisis in psychiatry means that it is increasingly rare for an assessment to be done by a senior clinician (the number of unfilled consultant posts has increased by 35% since 2017[4]). A homogenisation of standards is therefore necessary, and the bar is set at 'safe' rather than therapeutic. This was the problem that Camilla was facing. She already knew that she was safe, and had no intention of repeating the act of that day when her life fell apart. What she wanted was help in rebuilding her life. In this, she was thwarted by a system designed to avoid the worst-case scenario rather than helping patients feel better.

In the years since my appointment with Camilla, I saw first a trickle and then a steady stream of risk-related referrals. For patients, the cost of a risk being missed was obvious and devastating. For the psychiatrist, there was the psychological impact of such a tragedy happening to or being committed by someone you had been treating, but this was not even the worst of it. The sense of anguish was compounded by an increasing implication that the tragedy was avoidable. If something went wrong, then blame needed to be apportioned somewhere, and it was going to be your fault. These were the cases that led to the public shaming of doctors.

Homicide committed by someone because of severe mental illness is a devastating yet thankfully rare event (in the year ending March 2023, out of the 590 homicides committed in England and Wales, thirty-one were by someone with clear signs of mental illness[5]). During the 1990s though, lengthy reports were written in response to every case. The Latin phrase *post hoc ergo propter hoc* ('after this, therefore because of this') could have been coined for these 1990s homicide reports. In other words, if event B followed event A, it must be that event A caused event B. So, if a psychiatrist gave treatment X instead of treatment Y, and the patient came to harm, it was assumed that the treatment was responsible, and a different treatment would have led to a better outcome.

It doesn't take much thought to realise this logic is flawed, because it removes any agency from the individual patient and their choices. It also doesn't follow that an alternative drug or treatment plan would have changed anything. Yet the defining feature of the reports written around that time was that if something adverse happened to a patient, it could only mean that everything done to the patient, every interaction they'd had with psychiatric services, had brought them closer to the terrible tragedy being investigated. Little consideration was given to the range of events out of anyone's control that may have contributed – whether the patient had argued with their partner or friend, downed several pints of beer, decided to pay attention to a hallucination, felt threatened by a passer-by – all of these were secondary to the role played by the psychiatry team. Almost invariably, blame would be apportioned to the doctors, and sometimes also to the hospital trust or whoever else had been involved with the case. One such report all but finished the career of the psychiatrist who trained me as a medical student. I would stress that there's nothing wrong with wanting to understand what happened when there is a serious event like homicide, and how services might be improved to minimise the risks in the future, but blaming individuals for the failures of complex systems can be a way of avoiding looking at the deeper causes and feels symptomatic of a culture that thinks in terms of culpability rather than care.

It can be hard to imagine now how things used to be different, in the era before risk assessments. There was something about the richness of assessments that has been lost over the years. I recall a few years ago, I was asked to conduct a case review of a patient who, after many years of treatment, believed she had been misdiagnosed with schizophrenia. It was going to be a lot of extra work, and I didn't really have the time, but I agreed to do it because I generally believe that if it would be difficult to refuse, then it's best to accept with good grace. The notes arrived in a massive bundle: several volumes of written notes had yet to be archived onto the electronic notes system, and there were at least five more years' worth of notes in digital format on the hospital system. This was easily going to be a few days' work, to be squeezed around clinic appointments, phone calls, ward consultations and the variety of other jobs that made up my daily life. I dropped the first volume of notes onto my desk, where it landed with a thunk, and flipped open the first file. It dated back to the 1980s and detailed the patient's original contacts with mental health services, leading to the first of her many hospital admissions. Despite my initial reluctance to take on extra work, I soon got drawn into the case history.

Shola had just graduated from university and started an engineering graduate scheme job when she first saw a psychiatrist. Her behaviour had become erratic, arguing with the upstairs neighbours in her block of flats and accusing them of spying on her. Every time she walked into her flat, she could hear them upstairs in their flat in the exactly corresponding area. She felt this to be a subtle form of intimidation. 'Gaslighting' was not a term in common use then but would have described her perception that she was being tricked into thinking she was going mad.

In her frenetic evening hours, she had designed a new type of car engine to prove to her employers that despite the mental difficulties she was experiencing, they did not undermine her effectiveness as an employee. Tucked inside the notes was a thick sheet of folded paper. I pulled it out and saw it was the engine design. It was a detailed and complex drawing, and I couldn't make any sense of it. I carried on reading through the notes about the range of her symptoms, of paranoia and suspicion, and her delusional beliefs about her neighbours (she had by now moved flats, and a similar thing happened with her new neighbours – she was sure they had inserted cameras into each of the rooms in her house and were trying to control her with Bluetooth signals). Her thinking was becoming muddled, and the term 'thought disorder' was used in the notes, which described how her thoughts would become derailed, and her speech began to miss a logical flow to connect the ideas. By now, a fairly persuasive case was being built for the schizophrenia diagnosis she had questioned. I continued with the notes to see how things had played out over the years.

There was a lengthy, thoughtful entry from one of the junior doctors, committing himself to a diagnosis, and a diagnostic formulation to try to understand the psychological and social factors that may have contributed to her presentation. It was bold, because it allowed for the possibility of being wrong, and was written in a chatty and informal style that I found appealing. The next letter, though, stopped me in my tracks. It was a reply to the junior doctor from a firm of engineers. The doctor had actually sent the patient's engine design to the company to ask whether the engine might work, or whether this was the product of a disturbed mind. The firm politely expressed the view that the engine was unlikely to function. The doctor had shown an impressive wish to listen to and understand the patient's experience and a genuine interest and curiosity about her.

I returned to the patient's electronic notes a few days later to review the more recent entries. My shoulders sagged as I plodded through them. Nurses, doctors and therapists copied and pasted previous entries that described the diagnosis, followed by some brief account of the patient's interaction, which added little to the understanding of her mental experiences. (One journal article, looking at entries in electronic medical notes in a large US hospital between 2015 and 2020, depressingly showed that, by 2020, 54% of the text in electronic records had been copied and pasted from a previous entry, totalling over 16 billion words in the records reviewed during the study period.[6]) They all seemed to end with a remark that Shola was not at risk of suicide or homicide. There was little in the notes to make me question the original diagnosis of schizophrenia, but almost every time Shola was seen, she would have been questioned to establish her risk. I can't imagine what this question, asked by successive mental health professionals at her appointments, might have done to Shola's well-being or self-image. It can't have been long before she stopped seeing her own positive qualities, and started to define herself only in the negative – as the risk she may pose – because that's all anyone wanted to discuss.

At the inception of this preoccupation with forms, some in the profession could see it coming. A psychiatrist wrote an article in the *British Journal of Psychiatry* entitled 'Formarrhoea',[7] a word that nicely captured the unstoppable proliferation of forms. He described the increasingly bureaucratic approach to mental health care, in which, 'The standard of good practice will be a set of correctly-completed forms and followed procedures. Never mind how you and your patient actually get on.' He lamented 'the pressure to create risk-free public services, together with the belief that forms are the way to do it'.

A focus on risk also serves another purpose. In our current system of care, for a patient with schizophrenia admitted to an inpatient ward, the emphasis is on their stabilisation and discharge to free up hospital beds for the dozens of other patients waiting for that bed. Pressure on psychiatry inpatient beds is intense, with the number of beds for psychiatric inpatients in the UK falling from over 150,000 in the 1950s to about 27,000 by 2008.[8]

A more recent figure of 17,610 beds was reported for 2020–21.[9] A report commissioned by the Royal College of Psychiatrists in the UK showed bed occupancy of routinely over 90%.[10, 11] My experience has been that it is not uncommonly over 100%, because when a patient is given trial leave to see how they manage outside of a hospital, their bed is allocated to another patient. In this way, when a patient with schizophrenia is admitted to an inpatient ward, the decision to discharge them is often made on the basis of a risk assessment that shows low risk. Yet to actually reduce risk, what is needed is more intensive time and effort spent treating the patient properly, and assessing and managing their risk meaningfully. A more prolonged admission allows patients to enjoy a period of stability for the improvement to take hold, and for people to have the time to reintegrate back into normal life and have the best possible chance of avoiding a return stay. But extended admissions would bring psychiatry services grinding to a halt. There just isn't the capacity.

I remember as a junior doctor working for an old-school physician, the sort they don't make 'em like any more. I don't think I ever saw him out of his navy pinstripe suit, and he carried an air of unflappable calm. With his grey and thinning hair neatly combed into a side parting and his urbane manner and upper-class drawl, he inspired confidence and deference in even the most anxious or oppositional patients. Once he discovered that I was planning to switch from internal medicine to psychiatry, he treated me to his reflexively conservative views on mental health. It was a lengthy monologue, uninformed by evidence but deeply felt. The gist was that he 'didn't believe in it'. Yet the irony was that being 'old school', he took the time to listen to and engage with his patients, thereby providing them with a form of psychotherapy by another name.

I thought about him again years later whilst reading some academic papers on risk assessments. By now it was clear that trying to score a risk assessment, giving points for different answers and adding them up to provide a risk level, did little to mitigate risk and was potentially misleading. Before our preoccupation with risk became one of the central purposes of a psychiatric assessment, patient interactions and notes were routinely more colourful, rounded and therapeutic, just as Shola's had been. Over the years, many patient interactions have become formulaic, more impersonal and primarily interested in what is medically and legally defensible, should anything go wrong. The corollary of all of this is that people who really do want to get help from psychiatry services realise that if they play up their risk, services are more likely to respond. There is a belief that this is the only way to get care, which is not entirely wrong.

Psychiatry has always been, and will only ever be, about people. People like me and you, doing our best to navigate the turbulence and unpredictability of life. Occasionally our threshold is exceeded and our capacity to withstand what life has thrown at us starts to falter. Suicidal thoughts in the population are exceedingly common. One study, typical of many looking at general populations (rather than psychiatric populations) in Europe, showed that in Britain, at the time of the study, 7.4% of the population had suicidal thoughts.[12] In the US, a large population survey by the CDC put the overall figure at 4.3% having had suicidal thoughts during the preceding year.[13] Usually, these thoughts are in the abstract, a sense that life is too much to bear. People burdened by the cares of life often feel it would be easier if they didn't wake up in the morning. As the nineteenth-century American philosopher Henry David Thoreau famously said, 'The mass of men lead lives of quiet desperation.'

Risk assessment forms should really be seen as a series of prompts to engage in a conversation with the patient, rather than an end in themselves. In other words, to do what my physician colleague of yesteryear used to do, what psychiatrists come into the profession to do, and what the patients want and expect from us – to engage with them and their problems meaningfully in a way that does not involve using tick boxes or standardised questionnaires. This makes people feel more human, as if their lives and problems matter, and their hopes and thoughts are not considered a minor matter compared with the ever-present fear of something going wrong. Moving away from risk categories, and understanding and accepting the complexity and unpredictability of individuals should be the new normal. But this will need a greater investment in mental health services as well as the way care is delivered.

It is time to reverse the trend of decreasing inpatient bed numbers and to implement meaningful investment in psychiatry. At the moment, the lack of investment means that priority is given to the risky and dangerous. We need to be able to focus on what is important rather than what is urgent. This is the work that doesn't get measured. It is the quality of the patient interaction, the understanding of their lives and their personalities, as well as the thought and hard work that goes into making a meaningful diagnostic formulation and treatment plan. If we want to modify risk, we need to understand and value each person in our society. Not everything was better back in the old days, but the converse is also true – not every advance is progress.

13

Tomorrow's World

I've always had a soft spot for watching science fiction dramas, and how the future is imagined. There are hovering cars, precogs seeing into the future, mobile phone assistants that have gained sentience, and strangely tailored clothes. Health innovations are common too. Star Trek's system involved waving around a magic diagnostic stick, the tricorder, over the body of the sick or injured patient. The diagnosis would be rapidly revealed, and the treatment delivered by a device, the hypospray, that injected the curative substance directly into the body without using a needle. There would be a small 'psshhht' as the hypospray was pushed against the neck and the plunger pressed. It was how medicine was meant to be.

I often used to wonder how mental illness would be treated in the future. Generally, it was a topic ignored by science fiction writers. Inasmuch as it was covered in the Star Trek world, there were two broad approaches. The main theme seemed to be that mental illness was a quaint relic of a near-forgotten past, like money or petty ambition. I imagine the assumption was that the social utopia that led people to the stars also cured the world of mental illness. The second approach was the use of a telepathic, albeit human-looking woman from another planet, who could sense emotion and then offer counselling.

It struck me that there was a physical/mental health divide that even people with a free range to imagine the future couldn't get past. There were no tricorders to diagnose depression and differentiate it from the sadness of a missed Starfleet promotion. There were no little hisses of the hypospray to cure the onset of an obsessional disorder or the development of a psychotic breakdown that was being compounded by the terror of the infinite black depth of deep space.

Even if science fiction has failed to conjure a convincing future psychiatry, it is possible for us to draw on our knowledge of recent technological advances in physical medicine to imagine their application to conditions of the mind, understanding that mental problems originate or are marked within the brain. Where exactly though? Future technologies may have the answers. We may be able to follow thinking processes in the brain, to 'see' depression, anxiety and psychosis and prove that they are real and not, as some critics of psychiatry maintain, socially constructed artefacts.

There is an abundance of evidence that we can locate mental illness in the brain. Diseases such as Parkinson's disease and multiple sclerosis, for example, are well known to cause anxiety, depression and, less commonly, symptoms of psychosis. There is a branch of psychiatry known as immunopsychiatry that explores the effects of the immune system on the brain. In particular, it looks at how mental symptoms develop in response to the immune system having gone awry. To take one example, teratomas, which are tumours found in the ovaries in women, produce antibodies that affect the brain. These antibodies in some patients, amazingly, simulate the exact symptoms of schizophrenia. It would be an easy diagnosis to miss, not realising that the apparent schizophrenia is, in fact, caused by an ovarian tumour releasing antibodies. The ovaries are not an obvious place to look when someone is presenting with mental symptoms, but missing the diagnosis could be a disaster.[1]

When it comes to one of the most serious of mental illnesses, schizophrenia, autoimmune psychosis has been the focus of recent research. One study published in the *American Journal of Psychiatry* that examined a Danish nationwide register showed that autoimmune diseases developed in 3.6% of people with schizophrenia. Looking at it the other way round, 3.1% of people with auto-immune disease had a family history of schizophrenia.[2] These findings seem to be telling us something about the nature of mental illness and its interactions with the immune system. It ties in with a fact that has been in all the psychiatry textbooks for as long as I can remember. Schizophrenia is commoner in those born in winter, with an increased risk of about 5–15%.[3] A winter birthday is one of several risk factors for schizophrenia that can also affect the immune system, and who knows? Childhood abuse, racism, ostracism, social adversity – all these impact the immune system and therefore perhaps also the brain, further increasing the likelihood of schizophrenia.

The final piece of the jigsaw in understanding schizophrenia might come from genetic studies. We know that there is a significant genetic component in the development of schizophrenia. You might expect that a lot of this genetic risk relates to the genes that code for the brain, and that is true. Yet the biggest surprise, in a ground-breaking study published in *Nature*, was that many of the genes associated with schizophrenia play an important role in the immune system. Here is solid evidence that variations in the immune system may have an effect on brain function in schizophrenia, leading us closer to the scientific validation we are searching for.[4]

Yet a further problem remains. It's not enough to know that the brain is affected. The next question is how do we match up what is going wrong in the brain with what people tell us about their mental experiences? To give just one example, what does the statement 'I am sad' mean? At one level we understand what it means. Yet what are the brain processes that make someone have that thought, and can we ever find them? What actually is an emotion, and how can we relate that to brain receptors and cerebral function?

Computational psychiatry is a new area of research that is trying to answer these questions. It applies mathematical models to understand what the brain is doing at the detailed level of individual neurones and neuronal circuits. If we think of the healthy brain as performing countless computations, and we can describe these mathematically, it will allow us to better understand brain function in health. But perhaps more importantly, it may allow us to understand what is happening at the extremes of the distribution, the times when the brain is showing some signs of abnormality.

Consider, for example, panic attacks. If we imagine the brain as a dynamic system, then panic might be described as an example of a positive feedback loop that causes exponential growth, so that the panic just keeps on building. Other mental states may have different mathematical descriptions. When someone is stuck in a particular mood or way of thinking, it may be mathematically conceptualised as like a ball in a bowl. It keeps rolling back down to its default position, in the same way that people keep defaulting back to a mood state. Sometimes an individual reaches a state of what is known as critical slowing down, which precedes the transition from one mental state to another, a kind of tipping point. This may be modelled to show how people may enter into, or recover from, states of depression.

There are many other examples of how moods or behaviours can be described or predicted with computational modelling. These can lead to a more objective understanding of emotions and help us to identify brain dysfunction in emotion. The goal is that psychiatric diseases could be described in terms of a range of cellular dysfunctions that are linked together into networks, and this would give us a new framework for thinking about mental health and illness.

The computational approaches in psychiatry can lead to different ways of understanding other psychiatric symptoms. The brain is, in some respects, a machine that generates predictions about the world around us. It needs to manage uncertainty and errors in its predictions, based on the feedback it gets from the outside world. What happens when this process starts to go wrong? One fascinating experiment looked at models of hallucinations, and how these may be generated in the brain.[5] The researchers looked at both humans and mice. They played a pure tone in a noisy background, so that it was difficult to hear clearly. People were then asked if they heard the tone. In half the trials there was no tone, but a number of people were confident they had heard it. In effect, this was a hallucination – a confident report of hearing a tone that wasn't there. The people who 'heard' this tone were more prone to having spontaneous hallucinations (according to a pre-study questionnaire that asked about them) than those who didn't. Their prior expectations of what they expected to hear seemed to override their own sensory experience of what they were actually being played.

In the mouse part of the experiment, by administering ketamine, a substance known to increase hallucinations, mice were also more prone to 'hear' tones that weren't there (the experimenters had set up an elegant way of showing whether mice had heard a tone or not, based on the time they spent earning a reward). The researchers also found that manipulating dopamine in a particular part of the brain, an area thought to be central to hallucinations in schizophrenia, also increased the chance of mice having hallucinations. This effect was reversed by antipsychotic medication. In other words, by increasing activity in certain brain regions, our prior expectations of what we expect can override the reality of the world around us.

More speculatively, but along the same principles, consider the example of paranoia. Suppose my brain prediction is too heavily weighted towards the idea that people are plotting against me. As I walk down the street, I will start to observe the world around me. In my healthy state, I may conclude that my prediction is wrong. Everything is as it should be. The man in the house opposite is cleaning his car, the postman is walking down the street, and there is really no evidence that I am being watched. My brain will conclude that there is a prediction error. Its prediction, the prior expectation, is wrong based on the feedback it has received, and there is no reason to think people are plotting against me.

Yet what if my brain is in an unhealthy state? Random events in the environment are no longer filtered out. A bird tweeting in the tree may be sending signals. A traffic camera appears to glint in the sunlight as I walk by. My brain then weights these events. It sees that they support the original hypothesis that something bad is afoot. It has made an error in prediction that has not been corrected. In fact, it has been reinforced by random events in the environment, which have been given undue weight. My paranoia is intensified by my inability to filter out randomness, and in this way, the computations my brain is making lead me only further into mental illness.

The same process could be taking place in other emotional states, such as feeling hopeless. How does the brain decide how to assign a likelihood to certain beliefs being true, and how is it able to correct those beliefs in light of new information? Our brains are a way of allowing us to interact with our environment based on a huge amount of data, built up from prior experience, as well as our response to real-time feedback. If aspects of this system are failing, owing to faulty predictions and the inability to correct them, then mental illness may be the consequence.

Another way of trying to understand mental symptoms is in relation to machine learning, which is a promising branch of computational psychiatry. When we have very large data sets, we may be able to discern new patterns that we couldn't see before. This may allow us to see which symptoms that patients report cluster together. The way certain symptoms tend to cluster into groups may be telling us something about the underlying brain function and why we tend to see these symptoms together.

Recently, new classification systems for psychiatric symptoms based on these cluster models have been proposed. One such system has become known as HiTOP, which stands for Hierarchical Taxonomy of Psychopathology.[6] It views symptoms on a spectrum from normal to abnormal. It recognises that symptoms can cross diagnostic boundaries, so that symptoms of depression, for example, may overlap with those of other diagnoses like schizophrenia. At the moment, it is not in common use but it does suggest that our traditional way of looking at diagnosis in psychiatry is not all that there is, and that other ways of understanding diagnosis may be more accurate and represent something real that is happening inside the brain.

In psychiatry there are often hundreds or thousands of genes, each with a very small contribution but which cumulatively can increase the risk of developing a particular disease substantially. With large data sets of whole genomes, computational models may allow us to say which genes raise the risk of a certain illness. If we can work out what the genes do in the body, that too will give us an insight as to how mental illness develops.

Large data sets can potentially also allow us to predict things such as suicide risk. If we have enough data about who goes on to complete suicide, what their characteristics were and what sort of things they said, it may aid our ability to understand the risks an individual presents. Large data sets may also help us to predict which individuals are likely to respond to which medications. This might be correlated with the microscopic, for example, which drugs engage different neuronal processes (hopelessness, sadness, guilt), ushering in a new era of understanding the workings of the brain and precision psychiatry.

All of these developments point the way to a more personalised, accurate psychiatry, with the understanding of our neural pathways of emotion and the clustering of symptoms into diagnoses that correlate with what is going on in the brain. They may lead to the delivery of individualised treatments based on individual symptoms, metabolic pathways and genetics.

Of course, the usefulness of all these different possible tools in the understanding and treatment of mental illness will be dependent upon the humans who use them. As with symptom checklists or risk assessment forms, the readings from a genetic analysis or a data prediction require careful consideration in the context of the individual patient in front of you. And then there is the interpersonal factor. Consider what happens in a clinical interview between a psychiatrist and patient. Knowing what questions to ask is not hard to learn. Learning to listen carefully to the answers is a bit harder. If an AI device was shown hundreds of thousands of clinical interviews, listening to variations in voice, observing barely perceptible changes in facial expression and body language, would it then develop intuition? Is cumulative learning enough for AI to develop emotional rather than just logical intelligence? It is possible that AI could become a tool to assist clinicians in optimising performance. By processing a series of inputs about symptoms and aiding with diagnosis and treatment options, it may be a useful addition to the clinical process. But what of an 'intuition' about a patient? How do I know to ask this particular question at this moment, or to keep silent and let the patient reveal something they were not sure they were going to say? My belief is that this is one area in which the human connection will remain indispensable.

For now, many of these potential advances in psychiatry belong in a more distant future. In today's world, I think the biggest challenge is how we more clearly differentiate health and illness. Where are those bright lines that separate normal from abnormal? What validation can we bring to our diagnosis, in the same way that the rest of medicine has? Medicine has scans, blood tests, ECGs amongst a variety of ways to back up the doctor's diagnosis. Psychiatry has struggled to find a similar way of validating its diagnoses. It is a descriptive speciality, where diagnoses are still confirmed by identifying clusters of symptoms that form an overall pattern.

Descriptions matter, as do our assumptions behind them. These assumptions reflect the times we are living in and our current cultural moment, our shifting understanding of neurodiversity, and the individual experiences and different facets of ourselves that constitute our identity. All of these are shaping the conversation around mental health both culturally and clinically. The result is that we are now describing more of our normal human experiences as mental illnesses, or giving more of our individual variations in character and behaviour diagnostic labels. And whilst it is always important to look for underlying causes when rates of mental illness appear to be rising so sharply, I would contend that the starting point is to reconsider what counts as a psychiatric diagnosis.

Here I come back to a thought experiment from the Kendler paper[7] I talked about in Chapter 3. It's a question that keeps coming back to me. If we reran time again from the beginning, would we end up with the same psychiatric disorders? I think that certain core symptoms are unavoidably part of being human. In any world where there are people, we would have delusions, hallucinations and paranoia. Whether we would cluster these under the same umbrella and call them schizophrenia is less certain, but we would certainly see the same symptoms. There seem to be no societies where these symptoms of psychosis do not exist.

Similarly with the mood disorders, such as mania and depression, we would have the same euphoria in mania and the same sadness in depression, although I doubt we would describe the illnesses in exactly the same way, just as the current diagnoses have evolved around a core set of symptoms. Still, there would be something that looked like depression in our parallel world. The same would be true for anxiety disorders and obsessional disorders. I think again this would likely be the case throughout the world.

I would contend that for other diagnoses, they would likely not appear at all, or their characteristics would be thought of in a different way. Personality differences would emerge but may be understood as one of life's variations and not necessarily within the category of mental health problems. The same might be true of addictions, and even more so with behavioural addictions like sex addiction. I expect, too, that neurodevelopmental disorders would be understood differently in this parallel universe.

What counts as a mental disorder has sharply increased over the past seventy-five years. The first DSM manual of psychiatric disorders in 1952 (DSM-I) was 132 pages long, covering 128 categories. By 2013, DSM-5 had expanded to contain 541 categories, and at 947 pages[8] was 'thick enough to stop a bullet' according to a quote by one anonymous psychiatrist.[9] In other words, is there a core of mental illnesses, and are we able to identify them? It makes no logical sense that our progress through the past seventy-five years has only ever increased the number of diagnoses. The psychiatric profession has to take the lead in redrawing the diagnostic boundaries. I hope the next incarnation of DSM will start stripping back diagnoses rather than just adding to them. I would like to see tighter diagnostic guidelines. Not every variation of normal needs to be thought of as a diagnosable disorder. We also need to take a more robust view on lobbying by special interest groups and the pharmaceutical industry, and where there is doubt, to err on the side of excluding new diagnoses, whilst having a task force set up to remove ones that aren't working or aren't used.

Related to this is whether, for the diagnoses we do include, we can start to calibrate them more carefully. We have to find a way to ensure that diagnoses are robust entities, so they are only capturing mental illness and not variations of normal. Allen Frances, who chaired the DSM-IV task force, noted about anxiety, 'DSM-5 obscures the already fuzzy boundary between Generalized Anxiety Disorder and the worries of everyday life.'[10]

Even if we do reach a consensus on diagnostic categories, we also need to consider the increasingly divergent way in which diagnosis is thought about and used in the public discourse compared with how doctors use diagnosis. How do we move towards a position of respect for the patient's concerns and ideas about their diagnosis whilst acknowledging the clinician's expertise? We live in an age in which we no longer need to be automatically deferential to people and institutions. That is undoubtedly progress. Yet it has also brought us to a position of mistrust, including for mental healthcare. I think that as doctors we need to navigate this path, acknowledging our limitations whilst having confidence in our expertise. We need to be able to have sensible conversations both in our consultations and with the public about diagnoses, their basis, their boundaries and how they are made.

This will take some work. The language of mental health is everywhere, and it does not correlate with any standardised framework of mental illness. To further the confusion, we see the use of terms of health to describe illness. What does 'mental health' mean and how does it relate to 'mental illness'? It may not be possible to fully realign the professional and public understanding and expectations of what constitutes a mental health issue and what is a variation of normal, but adding the professional perspective back into the conversation is a start. This might also help redirect attention towards the underlying, structural pressures on mental health.

There are other factors we may be able to address in tackling the expansion of mental illness diagnoses. Over the past generation, there has increasingly been an atomisation of society. There are fewer formal rules and structures. We are not a religious society any longer, social structures are more fluid and there is a loss of community. There has been an increased number of people living alone.[11] Robert Putnam, in his article (and subsequent book) 'Bowling Alone', speaks of the loss of civic engagement in US society, using bowling as one example. He cites a figure of eighty million Americans who went bowling at least once in 1993. Yet whilst the number of people bowling in the US rose by 10% between 1980 and 1993, the number bowling in teams dropped by 40% over that same period.[12] It reflected something of the loss of community. Atomisation of societies and loneliness impact negatively on mental well-being,[13] and as clinicians we need to be aware of some of these reasons for increased mental illness, or perhaps increased identification with mental illness. The effects of atomisation of society, the demoralisation and feelings of being disconnected, can start to look like mental illness. In a busy clinic, when what appear to be symptoms of mental illness present to a doctor, they are often treated as such. But for many people, what appears to be depression or anxiety reflects a deeper lack of feeling valued, a sense of belonging and purpose.

Social prescribing may have a role in addressing this. For the younger generation, this may involve sports clubs, a local football team, youth centres. For others it might include painting, poetry, knitting, yoga, Pilates, sudoku, discussion groups, care farms. Walks in nature, even for as little as one hour, have been shown to reduce activity in stress-related brain regions.[14] For older people, being taught to use computers and smartphones can encourage agency. Taken together, these initiatives improve social interaction, social connection and confidence, and provide a sense of accomplishment. For those lacking it, they provide a structure to days and a sense of normality. All of these approaches can reduce symptoms that are often mistaken for those of mental illness, and the rates of mental illness themselves.

Having worked in psychiatry for nearly all of my professional life, I am deeply committed to the reality of psychiatric diagnosis and the importance of trying to define the essence of each particular illness. I believe that mental illness will ultimately be correlated with the abnormal workings of the brain. But for now, what we have is the expertise of those who have studied mental illness most closely and who have met and treated patients with a range of conditions. Psychiatry has always been set apart from other medical specialities, in part because the understanding of mental illness and the brain mechanisms that underlie it have been much harder to demonstrate. Cardiology might not be easy in practice, but everybody understands that the heart is an electrical pump that moves blood around the body; it is not conceptually difficult. Precisely because psychiatric illness has been so hard to pin down, people have tried to impose their own vision of what it is and what it represents.

We as a profession need to be confident in our expertise whilst being honest about the gaps in knowledge. Expertise has become unfashionable in recent years, but it takes time, training, judgement and care. The alternative has been the current position, of increasingly uncertain and self-defined illness, which comes at a real cost to the individual and to society. I fear the future backlash of a generation harmed by our passivity, and the accusation, 'You were meant to be the experts. Why didn't you say anything?'

14

Epilogue

It was one of those scorching hot afternoons in central London, where the air is still and the sounds of traffic and people walking by seem to hang in the sky. It was the sort of drowsy day that reminded me of childhood, summer holidays, the faint jingle of a distant ice cream van, of children's laughter. I was coming to the end of a long clinic. Chris was my final patient, and in the few minutes before I was due to see him, I reread my summary from his previous appointment. He was a thirty-nine-year-old man who had presented with symptoms of depression six weeks earlier. They were fairly typical symptoms, not the worst case I'd ever seen, but difficult enough for him. He was finding it hard to get through the day, lacking drive and motivation, and he had stopped going out aside from for work, where he was doing something in marketing. It had been a stressful time for him in his job though, with various reorganisations and job insecurity. More troubling to him, and what seemed to trigger the onset of his low mood, was his mother's death after a short illness about three months earlier. He was an only child and had been close to his mother, caring for her in her final weeks. And home wasn't much of a respite, where he had a young family including a hyperactive son. All in all, life was getting on top of him, and depression seemed to be the consequence. Our initial appointment came back to me as

I read the notes. I recalled a pleasant man, dressed in a dark suit and open-neck white shirt. He was someone you'd see on public transport and assume that nothing much was going wrong for him in life. He seemed stable and respectable, and his outward appearance didn't give any hint at his inner turmoil. In the end, after a bit of humming and hawing and discussion with him, I had started treatment with antidepressants.

I could see as soon as I stepped into the waiting room that he was much better. It was apparent in all those unmeasurable qualities of any doctor–patient interaction. He appeared lighter and chattier, laughed more easily, as we walked up the stairs to the consultation room. We sat down, and soon enough he told me how much better he was feeling. His days were a bit brighter, his sleep had improved and he had recovered some of his drive and motivation. He had booked to go on a summer holiday before the autumn term started, and was looking forward to a holiday in Greece with the family. There's nothing a doctor likes more than a patient getting better, and even more so at the end of a long clinical day. I was happy for the patient and pleased with myself for managing his care.

'So,' I said as I began to wrap the consultation up, 'any problems with the medication? Any side effects?'

'No, not really.'

'No?'

There was a pause. 'Well, I didn't actually take them in the end.'

'Oh,' I said, slightly disconcerted. 'What happened?'

'Well, I kept forgetting to pick up my prescription, then I went away for a weekend with my wife and started to feel better, so thought I'd try without tablets.'

Chris was just pleased to be feeling better, with not a hint of criticism about his care, yet I felt chastened. Chris's problems had been in that grey area where someone's symptoms may simply reflect the normal, everyday cares of life, or may be the harbingers of mental illness. It highlighted the danger of mistaking a normal emotional response for a pathological reaction.

I should have recognised that the key to Chris's case was his grief for his mother. Of all the many battlegrounds in the creation of DSM-5, none was quite so bitterly or publicly contested as the area of bereavement. Up to and including DSM-IV, there had been what was known as a 'bereavement exclusion' for depression. Put simply, the guidelines limited a diagnosis of depression if it came after a bereavement. As anyone who has been bereaved will know, there is a considerable overlap between grief and depression. There is the sadness, tearfulness, despair and sleepless nights, amongst a range of other emotions. The bereavement exclusion was in place to prevent depression being diagnosed when in reality the symptoms would have been a self-limiting reaction to the loss of a loved one. In other words, part of normal grief.

The decision in 2013 to remove the bereavement exclusion from DSM-5 provoked a storm of controversy. As one paper explained,[1] the authors of DSM-5 were unprepared for the avalanche of criticism that followed. They had seen it as a more technical change. Their argument was that many other things besides bereavement may trigger depression, such as work stresses, illness of someone close, divorce, and so forth, yet no exclusions are put into place for diagnosing depression that is triggered by any of those. So why should bereavement be any different?

I could hear the argument, but it was thin. The first point is that we don't diagnose depression in the context of any of those other things either. There is a category of diagnoses called 'adjustment disorders', which better describe that period of anxiety or sadness accompanying life's inevitable reversals and adversities. The implication of the diagnosis, and the reality for most, is that people do adjust to changes in circumstances, even if things can be emotionally quite rocky for a time. It is not that common to need to treat them. When I see people in these situations, perhaps after losing their job or a painful relationship breakup, some reassurance that such emotions are normal and common, and will usually pass without intervention, is enough for most people.

The second issue with the removal of the bereavement exclusion was that it had the potential to lead to even more depression being incorrectly diagnosed. We had already seen that with the expansion of diagnoses following DSM-IV. The chair of the task force for that iteration of DSM, psychiatrist Allen Frances, said that his biggest DSM-IV regret was 'broadening the autism definition that has led to such massive, careless over-diagnosis'.[2] But he also expressed deep concern over the removal of the bereavement exclusion,[3] no doubt fearing that if you give an inch, before you know it, you've given a mile. In fact, there already was a way to diagnose depression in bereavement if it was severe enough, so removing the exclusion merely opened the door to misdiagnosis, in which the sadness caused by grief might become recategorised as depression. Whereas previous DSM classifications might have stayed the hand of hard-pressed GPs and psychiatrists, the loosening of diagnostic boundaries, coupled with overenthusiastic pharmaceutical marketing, might contribute to the ever-expanding juggernaut of depression. In the event, that particular fear has not been borne out in the decade since DSM-5. There has been an expansion of antidepressant prescribing that feels increasingly out of control, but bereavement has not really been a part of that.

But there was another reason why people were so against the change to the bereavement exclusion, and why the popular press found it such a newsworthy story. The real objection was the medicalisation of grief. It was the feeling that something universally experienced, framed and understood throughout the centuries as part of religion, humanity and the rich tapestry of life was now being subject to a medical reductionism. People feared that they might not be seen as grieving but rather depressed. It seemed to represent something about the loss of values, perhaps even the loss of common sense.

One *Lancet* article[4] spoke of a cultural shift, what the author described as the 'infiltration of bureaucratic standards and regulations ever more deeply into ordinary life'. The spiritual, the ephemeral, was being brought into the prosaic business of diagnostic classification. The author, himself recently bereaved after forty-six years of marriage, felt by contrast that his grief and pain was part of his emergence into a new life. It served a purpose. It was not a troublesome irritation, like a fly that needed to be swatted away, or a hunger to be quickly satiated by a burger and chips. He saw meaning in his emotional pain, a spiritual connection, and the loss of this, the anaesthetising of the pain of grief, was not something to be readily embraced.

Similar sorts of discussions were had about the inclusion of prolonged or abnormal grief disorders in the newer revision of DSM-5. It presupposed that there is such a thing as a normal grief reaction. Yet not only is grief culturally influenced, it is also a very personal experience. One study[5] found that 34% of a large sample of bereaved individuals would meet the criteria for a prolonged grief disorder, particularly if it was a child or spouse that had died, or the death was from unnatural causes like suicide, homicide or overdose. More importantly though, most of the respondents did not think a diagnosis of prolonged grief disorder would be helpful to them. They mostly did not see their grief as being abnormal. Again, there is the intrusion of the state, of a bureaucratic classification, into the affairs of what many would consider everyday life. Whilst the opposing argument would be that such a diagnosis may allow people to access help and support, and have their problems formally acknowledged, this doesn't quite hold up, as help could

be accessed anyway without a formal diagnosis. There is no short-
age of bereavement charities and therapists who would be able to
offer guidance and support. The involvement of psychiatry in
grief feels largely unnecessary from a practical point of view, but
also more fundamentally. To grieve the loss of someone you have
known and loved is a normal response. This is what I should have
reminded Chris. It was what he, without knowing it, reminded me.

The life of any clinician is about making judgements. These
are often about treatments, their side effects, relative harms, the
risks and benefits. But the most fundamental judgement of all is in
delineating normal from abnormal health – who is ill and who is
not, who needs reassurance and who needs treatment. We should
save mental health care for those who need it. Life can be hard,
and the hard parts are unavoidable. But life's problems are a challenge to be overcome. Emotions are the natural consequence of
the struggles and triumphs, part of what gives life its variety, tex-
ture and meaning. These emotions may be disproportionate, or
even exaggerated or prolonged, but they are not necessarily a sign
of illness or disease. They are what make us human.

Acknowledgements

People think writing a book must be a solitary experience, and for a lot of time that is true. But I certainly couldn't have written this book alone. From the start and throughout, there has been the reassuring presence of my agent, Jonathan Conway, so wise, supportive and encouraging that without him I doubt that I could have got this book off the ground. It has also been a privilege to work with my wonderful editor, Laura Barber. From the very first meeting, I knew that she was the right person for me and for this book. Over time, I have only been able to admire the clarity of thought, intelligence and perceptiveness that she brought to the editorial process. The book has benefitted from her input in countless ways.

Trying to squeeze writing into a busy working life has not always been easy, and it was during the writing of this book that I rediscovered libraries. There has been my local library, where after two years I am now on nodding terms with the regulars. On Sundays there is the British Library and, whenever I have time, there is the Wellcome Library, perhaps the most beautiful of all libraries. I wanted to acknowledge here what an important and valuable resource the libraries in this country are.

I have had many conversations with colleagues throughout the writing of this book, and have been humbled by how generous people have been with their time. My neuropsychiatry colleagues Dr Tim Segal and Dr Simon Harrison deserve a special mention for all the many discussions, reading of drafts and insightful contributions they have made. Thanks too to the many other clinicians I spoke to, and discussed my ideas with and whose expertise I benefitted from. These include Prof. Dennis Ougrin, Dr Nigel Blackwood, Dr Renata Pires, Dr Mary Burgess, Prof. Guy Leschziner, Dr Stefanos Maltezos, Dr Sameer Jauhar, Dr Justin Sauer, Dr Tom Pollak and Dr Siobhan Gee. I am grateful too to Prof. Quentin Huys at UCL, Prof. Michael Sharpe in Oxford and Dr Awais Aftab in the US. And whilst I have tried to do justice to all the thoughtful comments and contributions from my colleagues, I would like to add that any errors in the book are mine alone.

I want to acknowledge my hospital, The South London and Maudsley NHS Foundation Trust, where I have worked now for almost thirty years and who have been such exemplary employers. I would also particularly like to thank the patients whom I have seen over the years, and for whom it has been a privilege to try to offer some help in difficult times.

Closer to home, I want to thank my sister, Kate Fulton, who has steadfastly remained my biggest cheerleader, and who was the first to read every chapter. Her feedback gave different perspectives on the book and helped give me the confidence to keep going. And to my brother Tim, and my in-laws, for all their support.

The support of family is what gives a stable base for any enterprise. To my wife Sara, who claimed only to have realised how much I love her when she got to the acknowledgement page of my last book, and who encouraged me to 'say something nice again' in the acknowledgements this time – perhaps as a psychiatrist I could be a little more expressive, but my love for you remains undiminished. And to our four boys, now all grown up, who make me proud every day.

Finally to my parents. Whilst I was writing this book, my father had a stroke and has been in a nursing home since. He was a lawyer but always held the medical profession in such high esteem, so for as long as I can remember, he encouraged me to do medicine. My mother too has always enjoyed having a son as a doctor, and even now will come to me first with any health complaint (Mum, I'm a psychiatrist). Thank you both for everything you gave me. This book is dedicated to you.

Notes

1. Introduction

1   Majority of students experience mental health issues, says NUS survey. *Guardian*. 14 December 2015. https://www.theguardian. com/education/2015/dec/14/majority-of-students-experience-mental-health-issues-says-nus-survey

2   NUS survey finds students experience mental health issues. Open Access Government. 15 December 2015. https://www. openaccessgovernment.org/nus-survey-finds-students-experience-mental-health-issues/23255/

3   Arie S. 'Simon Wessely: Every time we have a mental health awareness week my spirits sink'. *BMJ*. 2017;358. doi:10.1136/bmj. j4305

4   Russell G, Stapley S, Newlove-Delgado T, et al. Time trends in autism diagnosis over 20 years: a UK population-based cohort study. *J Child Psychol Psychiatry*. 2022;63(6):674–682. doi:10.1111/jcpp.13505

5   Blashfield RK, Keeley JW, Flanagan EH, Miles SR. The cycle of classification: DSM-I through DSM-5. *Annu Rev Clin Psychol*. 2014;10:25–51. doi:10.1146/annurev-clinpsy-032813-153639

6   What we know about the UK's working-age health challenge. The Health Foundation. 17 November 2023. https://www.health. org.uk/publications/long-reads/what-we-know-about-the-uk-s-working-age-health-challenge

7   Mental health. World Health Organization. 17 June 2022. https:// www.who.int/news-room/fact-sheets/detail/mental-health-strengthening-our-response

8   Westerhof GJ, Keyes CLM. Mental illness and mental health: the two continua model across the lifespan. *J Adult Dev*. 2010;17(2):110–119. doi:10.1007/s10804-009-9082-y

9   Mental health apps market size, share & trends analysis report by
         platform (Android, iOS), by application (meditation management,
         stress management), by region, and segment forecasts, 2024–2030.
         Grand View Research. Accessed 10 March 2024. https://www.
         grandviewresearch.com/industry-analysis/mental-health-apps-
         market-report

10   Gerber L, Gaudillière JP. Marketing masked depression: physicians,
         pharmaceutical firms, and the redefinition of mood disorders in the
         1960s and 1970s. *Bull Hist Med*. 2016;90(3):455–490. doi:10.1353/
         bhm.2016.0073

11   How to stop over-medicalising mental health. *The Economist*.
         7 December 2023. https://www.economist.com/leaders/
         2023/12/07/how-to-stop-over-medicalising-mental-health

2. Psychiatry and Antipsychiatry

1   Scull A. *Madness in Civilization: A Cultural History of Insanity, from
         the Bible to Freud, from the Madhouse to Modern Medicine*. Thames &
         Hudson, 2015, pp. 26–28.

2   Hajar R. The air of history (part II) medicine in the Middle Ages.
         Heart Views. 2012;13(4):158. doi:10.4103/1995-705X.105744

3   Donzé PY, Fernández Pérez P. Health industries in the twentieth
         century. *Bus Hist*. 2019;61(3):385–403. doi:10.1080/00076791.201
         9.1572116

4   Houston RA. Asylums: the historical perspective before, during,
         and after. *Lancet Psychiatry*. 2020;7(4):354–362. doi:10.1016/S2215-
         0366(19)30395-5

5   Ban TA. Fifty years chlorpromazine: a historical perspective.
         Neuropsychiatr Dis Treat. 2007;3(4):495. https://www.ncbi.nlm.nih.
         gov/pmc/articles/PMC2655089/

6   Hillhouse TM, Porter JH. A brief history of the development of
         antidepressant drugs: from monoamines to glutamate. *Exp Clin
         Psychopharmacol*. 2015;23(1):1. doi:10.1037/A0038550

7   Powell E. Speeches of John Enoch Powell. enochpowell.info. 2011.
         http://enochpowell.info/wp-content/uploads/Speeches/June-
         Oct%201968.pdf

8   Goffman E. *Asylums: Essays on the Social Situation of Mental Patients
         and Other Inmates*. Anchor Books, 1961.

9   Szasz TS. The myth of mental illness. *Am Psychol*. 1960;15(2):113–118. doi:10.1037/h0046535

10   Berlim MT, Fleck MPA, Shorter E. Notes on antipsychiatry. *Eur Arch Psychiatry Clin Neurosci*. 2003;253(2):61–67. doi:10.1007/s00406-003-0407-8

11   Harrington A. The fall of the schizophrenogenic mother. *Lancet*. 2012;379(9823):1292–1293. doi:10.1016/S0140-6736(12)60546-7

12   Johnston J. The ghost of the schizophrenogenic mother. *AMA J Ethics*. 2013;15(9):801–805. doi:10.1001/virtualmentor.2013.15.9.oped1-1309

13   Rosenhan DL. On being sane in insane places. *Science*. 1973;179(4070):250–258. doi:10.1126/science.179.4070.250

14   Spitzer RL. On pseudoscience in science, logic in remission, and psychiatric diagnosis: a critique of Rosenhan's 'On Being Sane in Insane Places'. *J Abnorm Psychol*. 1975;84(5):442–452. doi:10.1037/h0077124

15   Scull A. Rosenhan revisited: successful scientific fraud. *Hist Psychiatry*. 2023;34(2):180–195. doi:10.1177/0957154X221150878

16   McDonald WM, Weiner RD, Fochtmann LJ, McCall WV. The FDA and ECT. *J ECT*. 2016;32(2):75–77. doi:10.1097/YCT.0000000000000326

17   Ayoub SS. (2021). Paracetamol (acetaminophen): a familiar drug with an unexplained mechanism of action. *Temperature*. 2021:8(4);351–371. doi:10.1080/23328940.2021.1886392

18   Son Y. Molecular mechanisms of general anesthesia. *Korean J Anesthesiol*. 2010;59(1):3–8. doi:10.4097/kjae.2010.59.1.3

19   Johnstone L, Boyle M, With Cromby J, Dillon J, Harper D, Longden P. The Power Threat Meaning Framework: Overview. January 2018. https://cms.bps.org.uk/sites/default/files/2022-07/PTM%20Framework%20%28January%202018%29_0.pdf

20   Ross M. The truth behind U of T's anti-psychiatry scholarship. *Huffington Post*. 17 October 2016. https://www.huffpost.com/archive/ca/entry/the-truth-behind-u-of-ts-anti-psychiatry-scholarship_b_12473034

3. A Diagnostic Dilemma

1   David AS, Nicholson T. Are neurological and psychiatric disorders different? *Br J Psychiatry J Ment Sci*. 2015;207(5):373–374. doi:10.1192/bjp.bp.114.158550

2   Kendler KS. The nature of psychiatric disorders. *World Psychiatry*.
        2016;15(1):5–12. doi:10.1002/wps.20292

3   Borsboom D. Psychometric perspectives on diagnostic systems.
        J Clin Psychol. 2008;64(9):1089–1108. doi:10.1002/jclp.20503

4   Zachar P, Kendler KS. A diagnostic and statistical manual of mental
        disorders history of premenstrual dysphoric disorder. *J Nerv Ment
        Dis*. 2014;202(4). doi:10.1097/nmd.0000000000000128

5   Scull A. *Hysteria: The Biography*. Oxford University Press, 2009, p. 13.

6   Schroll JB, Lauritsen MP. Premenstrual dysphoric disorder:
        A controversial new diagnosis. *Acta Obstet Gynecol Scand*.
        2022;101(5):482–483. doi:10.1111/aogs.14360

7   Yonkers KA, Simoni MK. Premenstrual disorders. *Am J Obstet
        Gynecol*. 2018;218(1):68–74. doi:10.1016/j.ajog.2017.05.045

8   Haslam N. Looping effects and the expanding concept of mental
        disorder. *Lang Ment Disord J Psychopathol*. 2016;22:4–9. https://old.
        jpsychopathol.it/wp-content/uploads/2016/02/02_Art_INTRO_
        Haslan1.pdf

9   Lindholm SK, Wickström A. 'Looping effects' related to young
        people's mental health: how young people transform the meaning
        of psychiatric concepts. *Glob Stud Child*. 2020;10(1):26–38.
        doi:10.1177/2043610619890058

10   Foulkes L, Andrews JL. Are mental health awareness efforts
        contributing to the rise in reported mental health problems?
        A call to test the prevalence inflation hypothesis. *New Ideas
        Psychol*. 2023;69:101010. https://doi.org/10.1016/j.
        newideapsych.2023.101010

11   The four principles of medical ethics. Medical Protection. 8
        February 2024. https://www.medicalprotection.org/uk/articles/
        essential-learning-law-and-ethics

12   Boyle CM. Difference between patients' and doctors' interpretation
        of some common medical terms. *BMJ*. 1970;2(5704):286–289.
        doi:10.1136/bmj.2.5704.286

13   Weinman J, Yusuf G, Berks R, Rayner S, Petrie KJ. How accurate
        is patients' anatomical knowledge: a cross-sectional, questionnaire
        study of six patient groups and a general public sample. *BMC Fam
        Pract*. 2009;10(1):43. doi:10.1186/1471-2296-10-43

14   Kahneman D. *Thinking, Fast and Slow*. Ebook edition.
        Penguin, 2011

15   Factors influencing COVID-19 vaccine uptake among minority
      ethnic groups. GOV.UK. 17 December 2000. https://www.gov.uk/
      government/publications/factors-influencing-covid-19-vaccine-
      uptake-among-minority-ethnic-groups-17-december-2020

4. Memories

1   Sulin RA, Dooling DJ. Intrusion of a thematic idea in retention of
      prose. *J Exp Psychol.* 1974;103:255–262. doi:10.1037/h0036846
2   How eyewitness misidentification can send innocent people to
      prison. Innocence Project. 15 April 2020. https://innocenceproject.
      org/how-eyewitness-misidentification-can-send-innocent-people-
      to-prison/
3   Ofshe R, Watters E. *Making Monsters: False Memories, Psychotherapy,
      and Sexual Hysteria.* University of California Press, 1996.
4   Brewin CR, Andrews B. Recovered memories of trauma:
      phenomenology and cognitive mechanisms. *Clin Psychol Rev.*
      1998;18(8):949–970. doi:10.1016/S0272-7358(98)00040-3
5   Bourget D, Gagné P, Wood SF. Dissociation: defining the
      concept in criminal forensic psychiatry. *J Am Acad Psychiatry
      Law.* 2017;45(2):147–160. https://www.researchgate.net/
      publication/381769335_Dissociation_Defining_the_Concept_in_
      Criminal_Forensic_Psychiatry
6   Merckelbach H, Christiansen SÅ. Amnesia for homicide as a form of
      malingering. In Christiansen SÅ (ed.). *Offenders' Memories of Violent
      Crimes.* John Wiley & Sons, Ltd., 2007, pp. 165–190. https://www.
      haraldmerckelbach.nl/artikelen_engels/2007/Amnesia%20For%20
      Homicide%20As%20A%20Form%20Of%20Malingering.pdf
7   McWhirter L, Ritchie C, Stone J, Carson A. Functional cognitive
      disorders: a systematic review. *Lancet Psychiatry.* 2020;7(2):191–207.
      doi:10.1016/s2215-0366(19)30405-5
8   Cabreira V, Frostholm L, McWhirter L, Stone J, Carson A. Clinical
      signs in functional cognitive disorders: a systematic review and
      diagnostic meta-analysis. *J Psychosom Res.* 2023;173:111447.
      doi:10.1016/j.jpsychores.2023.111447
9   Broshek DK, De Marco AP, Freeman JR. A review of post-
      concussion syndrome and psychological factors associated with
      concussion. *Brain Inj.* 2015;29(2):228–237. doi:10.3109/02699052.
      2014.974674

10   Mittenberg W, DiGiulio DV, Perrin S, Bass AE. Symptoms following
        mild head injury: expectation as aetiology. *J Neurol Neurosurg
        Psychiatry*. 1992;55(3):200–204. doi:10.1136/jnnp.55.3.200

11   Foster JS, Kenneth R. We don't need to choose between brain
        injury and 'mass hysteria' to explain Havana syndrome. *Scientific
        American*. 22 May 2024. https://www.scientificamerican.com/
        article/havana-syndrome-we-dont-need-to-choose-between-brain-
        injury-and-mass/

12   1990: 'Guinness Four' guilty. *BBC News*. Accessed 26 March 2024.
        http://news.bbc.co.uk/onthisday/hi/dates/stories/august/27/
        newsid_2536000/2536035.stm

13   Profile: Ernest Saunders; out of jail and back in business.
        Independent. 17 May 1996. https://www.independent.co.uk/voices/
        profile-ernest-saunders-out-of-jail-and-back-in-business-1347932.
        html

14   Howard R, Lovestone S, Levy R. Ernest Saunders: diagnostic
        dilemma. *Br Med J*. 1992;304(6841):1568. doi:10.1136/
        BMJ.304.6841.1568-A

15   Lacorte E, Ancidoni A, Zaccaria V, et al. Safety and efficacy of
        monoclonal antibodies for Alzheimer's disease: a systematic review
        and meta-analysis of published and unpublished clinical trials. *J
        Alzheimers Dis*. 2022;87(1):101–129. doi:10.3233/JAD-220046

5. Schizophrenia

1   Wilkinson G. Political dissent and 'sluggish' schizophrenia in the
        Soviet Union. *Br Med J Clin Res Ed*. 1986;293(6548):641–642.
        doi:10.1136/bmj.293.6548.641

2   van Voren R. Political abuse of psychiatry—an historical overview.
        Schizophr Bull. 2009;36(1):33–35. doi:10.1093/schbul/sbp119

3   Merskey H, Shafran B. Political hazards in the diagnosis of 'sluggish
        schizophrenia'. *Br J Psychiatry*. 1986;148:247–256. doi:10.1192/
        bjp.148.3.247

4   Ougrin D, Gluzman S, Dratcu L. Psychiatry in post-communist
        Ukraine: dismantling the past, paving the way for the future.
        Psychiatr Bull. 2006;30(12):456–459. doi:10.1192/pb.30.12.456

5   Charlson FJ, Ferrari AJ, Santomauro DF, et al. Global epidemiology
        and burden of schizophrenia: findings from the global burden of

disease study 2016. *Schizophr Bull.* 2018;44(6):1195. doi:10.1093/SCHBUL/SBY058

6   Moritz S, Gawęda Ł, Carpenter WT, et al. What Kurt Schneider really said and what the DSM has made of it in its different editions: a plea to redefine hallucinations in schizophrenia. *Schizophr Bull.* 2024;50(1):22–31. doi:10.1093/schbul/sbad131

7   Mitchell J, Vierkant AD. Delusions and hallucinations as a reflection of the subcultural milieu among psychotic patients of the 1930s and 1980s. *J Psychol.* 1989;123(3):269–274. doi:10.1080/00223980.1989.10542981

8   Ohayon MM, Priest RG, Caulet M, Guilleminault C. Hypnagogic and hypnopompic hallucinations: pathological phenomena? *Br J Psychiatry.* 1996;169(4):459–467. doi:10.1192/bjp.169.4.459

9   Larøi F, Luhrmann TM, Bell V, et al. Culture and hallucinations: overview and future directions. *Schizophr Bull.* 2014;40(4):213–220. doi:10.1093/schbul/sbu012

10 Barrett RJ. Kurt Schneider in Borneo: do first rank symptoms apply to the Iban? In: Jenkins JH, Barrett RJ, eds. *Schizophrenia, Culture, and Subjectivity: The Edge of Experience.* Cambridge Studies in Medical Anthropology. Cambridge University Press, 2003, pp. 87–109. doi:10.1017/CBO9780511616297.006

11 Okafor IP, Oyewale DV, Ohazurike C, Ogunyemi AO. Role of traditional beliefs in the knowledge and perceptions of mental health and illness amongst rural-dwelling women in western Nigeria. *Afr J Primary Health Care Fam Med.* 2022;14(1):e1–e8. doi:10.4102/phcfm.v14i1.3547

12 Padma TV. Developing countries: the outcomes paradox. *Nature.* 2014;508(7494):S14–S15. doi:10.1038/508S14a

13 Leff J, Vaughn C. The role of maintenance therapy and relatives' expressed emotion in relapse of schizophrenia: a two-year follow-up. *Br J Psychiatry.* 1981;139(2):102–104. doi:10.1192/bjp.139.2.102

6. The Evolution of Depression

1   Griffin E, McMahon E, McNicholas F, Corcoran P, Perry IJ, Arensman E. Increasing rates of self-harm among children, adolescents and young adults: a 10-year national registry study 2007-2016. *Soc Psychiatry Psychiatr Epidemiol.* 2018;53(7):663–671. doi:10.1007/s00127-018-1522-1

2   Horwitz AV, Wakefield JC, Lorenzo-Luaces L. History of depression.
        In DeRubeis RJ, Strunk DR (eds.). *The Oxford Handbook of Mood
        Disorders*. Oxford University Press, 2017, pp. 11–23.

3   Patel RK, Rose GM. Persistent depressive disorder. In: *StatPearls*.
        StatPearls Publishing, 2024. http://www.ncbi.nlm.nih.gov/books/
        NBK541052/

4   Goodwin RD, Dierker LC, Wu M, Galea S, Hoven CW, Weinberger
        AH. Trends in U.S. depression prevalence from 2015 to 2020:
        the widening treatment gap. *Am J Prev Med*. 2022;63(5):726.
        doi:10.1016/J.AMEPRE.2022.05.014

5   Brown GW, Harris TO. *Social Origins of Depression: A Study of
        Psychiatric Disorder in Women*. The Free Press, 1978.

6   Marsh C. Order and place in England, 1580–1640: the view from
        the pew. *J Br Stud*. 2005;44(1):3–26. doi:10.1086/424947

7   Graeber D, Wengrow D. *The Dawn of Everything: A New History of
        Humanity*. Farrar, Straus and Giroux, 2021. https://books.google.
        co.uk/books?id=9xkQEAAAQBAJ

8   Did disabled workers enjoy greater rights in centuries past?
        BBC News. 26 June 2014. https://www.bbc.co.uk/news/blogs-
        ouch-27975766

9   Frankl VE. *Man's Search for Meaning*. Simon and Schuster, 1984.

10   Paykel ES, Hart D, Priest RG. Changes in public attitudes to
        depression during the Defeat Depression Campaign. *Br J Psychiatry*.
        1998;173:519–522. doi:10.1192/bjp.173.6.519

11   Kendler KS. The phenomenology of major depression and the
        representativeness and nature of DSM criteria. *Am J Psychiatry*.
        2016;173(8):771–780. doi:10.1176/appi.ajp.2016.15121509

12   Cassel CK, Guest JA. Choosing wisely: helping physicians
        and patients make smart decisions about their care. *JAMA*.
        2012;307(17):1801–1802. doi:10.1001/jama.2012.476

13   Rosenthal NE, Sack DA, Gillin JC, et al. Seasonal affective disorder:
        a description of the syndrome and preliminary findings with light
        therapy. *Arch Gen Psychiatry*. 1984;41(1):72–80. doi:10.1001/
        archpsyc.1984.01790120076010

14   Traffanstedt MK, Mehta S, LoBello SG. Major depression
        with seasonal variation: is it a valid construct? *Clin Psychol Sci*.
        2016;4(5):825–834. doi:10.1177/2167702615615867

15   Young MA. Does seasonal affective disorder exist? A commentary

on Traffanstedt, Mehta, and LoBello (2016). *Clin Psychol Sci.* 2017;5(4):750–754. doi:10.1177/2167702616689086

16   Winthorst WH, Bos EH, Roest AM, de Jonge P. Seasonality of mood and affect in a large general population sample. *PLOS ONE.* 2020;15(9):e0239033. doi:10.1371/journal.pone.0239033

17   Magnusson A, Axelsson J, Karlsson MM, Oskarsson H. Lack of seasonal mood change in the Icelandic population: results of a cross-sectional study. *Am J Psychiatry.* 2000;157(2):234–238. doi:10.1176/appi.ajp.157.2.234

18   LoBello SG, Mehta S. No evidence of seasonal variation in mild forms of depression. *J Behav Ther Exp Psychiatry.* 2019;62:72–79. doi:10.1016/j.jbtep.2018.09.003

19   Nussbaumer-Streit B, Forneris CA, Morgan LC, et al. Light therapy for preventing seasonal affective disorder. *Cochrane Database Syst Rev.* 2019;3(3):CD011269. doi:10.1002/14651858.CD011269. pub3

20   Kendler KS. The nature of psychiatric disorders. *World Psychiatry.* 2016;15(1):5–12. doi:10.1002/wps.20292

21   Melrose S. Seasonal affective disorder: an overview of assessment and treatment approaches. *Depress Res Treat.* 2015;2015:178564. doi:10.1155/2015/178564

22   Iacobucci G. NHS prescribed record number of antidepressants last year. *BMJ.* 2019;364. doi:10.1136/bmj.l1508

23   Antidepressant prescriptions in England double in a decade. *Guardian.* 29 March 2019. https://www.theguardian.com/ society/2019/mar/29/antidepressant-prescriptions-in-england- double-in-a-decade

24   Fournier JC, DeRubeis RJ, Hollon SD, et al. Antidepressant drug effects and depression severity: a patient-level meta-analysis. *JAMA.* 2010;303(1):47–53. doi:10.1001/jama.2009.1943

25   Saxon D, Firth N, Barkham M. The relationship between therapist effects and therapy delivery factors: therapy modality, dosage, and non-completion. *Adm Policy Ment Health.* 2017;44(5):705–715. doi:10.1007/s10488-016-0750-5

7. Traumatised

1   Jones E, Wessely S. A paradigm shift in the conceptualization of psychological trauma in the 20th century. *J Anxiety Disord.* 2007;21(2):164–175. doi:10.1016/J.JANXDIS.2006.09.009

2   Efstratiou S. Introduction of the term 'trauma' in psychiatry.
         Ann Gen Psychiatry. 2010;9(1):S235. doi:10.1186/1744-859X-9-
         S1-S235

3   Lerner P, Micale MS. Trauma, psychiatry, and history: a conceptual
         and historiographical introduction. In Micale MS, Lerner P
         (eds.). *Traumatic Pasts: History, Psychiatry, and Trauma in the Modern
         Age, 1870–1930*. Cambridge Studies in the History of Medicine.
         Cambridge University Press, 2001, pp. 1–28. doi:10.1017/
         CBO9780511529252.002

4   Scull A. *Hysteria: The Biography*. Oxford University Press, 2009,
         pp. 104–130.

5   Jones E, Wessely S. Psychological trauma: a historical perspective.
         Psychiatry. 2006;5(7):217–220. https://doi.org/10.1053/j.
         mppsy.2006.04.011

6   Shell shock 1922. The National Archives. 1922. https://www.
         nationalarchives.gov.uk/wp-content/uploads/2018/11/wo32-4748.jpg

7   Stellman JM, Stellman SD, Sommer Jr JF. Social and behavioral
         consequences of the Vietnam experience among American
         Legionnaires. *Environ Res*. 1988;47(2):129–149. doi:10.1016/s0013-
         9351(88)80038-0

8   Jones E, Vermaas RH, McCartney H, et al. Flashbacks and post-
         traumatic stress disorder: the genesis of a 20th-century diagnosis. *Br
         J Psychiatry*. 2003;182(2):158–163. doi:10.1192/bjp.182.2.158

9   *Diagnostic and Statistical Manual of Mental Disorders (3rd Ed.)*.
         American Psychiatric Association, 1980.

10   Rose SC, Bisson J, Churchill R WS. Psychological debriefing for
         preventing post traumatic stress disorder (PTSD). *Cochrane Database
         Syst Rev*. 2002:(2):CD000560. doi:10.1002/14651858.CD000560

11   Rubin GJ, Brewin CR, Greenberg N, Simpson J, Wessely S.
         Psychological and behavioural reactions to the bombings in
         London on 7 July 2005: cross sectional survey of a representative
         sample of Londoners. *BMJ*. 2005;331(7517):606. doi:10.1136/
         BMJ.38583.728484.3A

12   Stramaccia DF, Meyer AK, Rischer KM, Fawcett JM, Benoit RG.
         Memory suppression and its deficiency in psychological disorders:
         A focused meta-analysis. *J Exp Psychol Gen*. 2021;150(5):828.
         doi:10.1037/xge0000971

13   McCormack K. Sharon Osbourne breaks silence after Sheryl

Underwood's PTSD claims on The Talk. *The Mirror*. 13 April 2021. https://www.mirror.co.uk/tv/tv-news/sharon-osbourne-breaks-silence-after-23907114

14   Loftus EF, Palmer JC. Reconstruction of automobile destruction: an example of the interaction between language and memory. *J Verbal Learn Verbal Behav*. 1974;13(5):585–589. doi:10.1016/S0022-5371(74)80011-3

15   Bridgland VME, Jones PJ, Bellet BW. A meta-analysis of the efficacy of trigger warnings, content warnings, and content notes. *Clin Psychol Sci*. 2023:12(4). doi:10.1177/21677026231186625

16   Jones PJ, Bellet BW, McNally RJ. Helping or harming? The effect of trigger warnings on individuals with trauma histories. *Clin Psychol Sci*. 2020;8(5):905–917. doi:10.1177/2167702620921341

17   Landin-Romero R, Moreno-Alcazar A, Pagani M, Amann BL. How does eye movement desensitization and reprocessing therapy work? A systematic review on suggested mechanisms of action. *Front Psychol*. 2018;9. doi:10.3389/fpsyg.2018.01395

8. The Rise (and Rise) of Neurodevelopmental Disorders

1   Duty calls. xkcd. Accessed 22 September 2024. https://xkcd.com/386/

2   dougbratton.com. Accessed 18 October 2024. http://www.dougbratton.com/comics.html

3   Layton TJ, Barnett ML, Hicks TR, Jena AB. Attention deficit–hyperactivity disorder and month of school enrollment. *N Engl J Med*. 2018;379(22):2122–2130. doi:10.1056/NEJMoa1806828

4   Faraone SV, Biederman J, Mick E. The age-dependent decline of attention deficit hyperactivity disorder: a meta-analysis of follow-up studies. *Psychol Med*. 2006;36(2):159–165. doi:10.1017/S003329170500471X

5   Eight-year ADHD backlog in many parts of UK, BBC finds. *BBC News*. 24 July 2024. https://www.bbc.com/news/articles/c720r1pxrx5o

6   BBC One. *Panorama*, 'Private ADHD Clinics Exposed'. 20 May 2023. https://www.bbc.co.uk/programmes/m001m0f9

7   Moffitt TE, Houts R, Asherson P, et al. Is adult ADHD a childhood-onset neurodevelopmental disorder? Evidence from a four-decade

longitudinal cohort study. *Am J Psychiatry*. 2015;172(10):967–977. doi:10.1176/appi.ajp.2015.14101266

8   Symptoms attention deficit hyperactivity disorder. NHS. Accessed 4 July 2023. https://www.nhs.uk/conditions/attention-deficit-hyperactivity-disorder-adhd/symptoms/

9   Paris J, Bhat V, Thombs B. Is adult attention-deficit hyperactivity disorder being overdiagnosed? *Can J Psychiatry*. 2015;60(7):324–328. doi:10.1177/070674371506000705

10   ADHD throughout the years. Centers for Disease Control and Prevention. 15 May 2024. https://www.cdc.gov/adhd/data/adhd-throughout-the-years.html?CDC_AAref_Val=https://www.cdc.gov/ncbddd/adhd/timeline.html

11   Kessler RC, Adler L, Barkley R, et al. The prevalence and correlates of adult ADHD in the United States: results from the National Comorbidity Survey Replication. *Am J Psychiatry*. 2006;163(4):716–723. doi:10.1176/ajp.2006.163.4.716

12   Frances A. *Saving Normal: An Insider's Revolt Against Out-of-control Psychiatric Diagnosis, DSM-5, Big Pharma and the Medicalization of Ordinary Life*. Ebook edition. Mariner Books, 2013.

13   Das S, Ungoed-Thomas J. Revealed: drug firms funding UK patient groups that lobby for NHS approval of medicines. *Observer*. 22 July 2023. https://www.theguardian.com/science/2023/jul/22/revealed-drug-firms-funding-uk-patient-groups-that-lobby-for-nhs-approval-of-medicines

14   Beau-Lejdstrom R, Douglas I, Evans SJW, Smeeth L. Latest trends in ADHD drug prescribing patterns in children in the UK: prevalence, incidence and persistence. *BMJ Open*. 2016;6(6):e010508. doi:10.1136/bmjopen-2015-010508

15   Avin MM, Teeling M, Bennett KE. Trends in attention-deficit and hyperactivity disorder (ADHD) medications among children and young adults in Ireland: a repeated cross-sectional study from 2005 to 2015. *BMJ Open*. 2020;10(4):e035716. doi:10.1136/bmjopen-2019-035716

16   Raman SR, Man KKC, Bahmanyar S, et al. Trends in attention-deficit hyperactivity disorder medication use: a retrospective observational study using population-based databases. *Lancet Psychiatry*. 2018;5(10):824–835. doi:10.1016/S2215-0366(18)30293-1

17   Tucha L, Fuermaier ABM, Koerts J, Groen Y, Thome J. Detection

of feigned attention deficit hyperactivity disorder. *J Neural Transm.* 2015;122(1):123–134. doi:10.1007/s00702-014-1274-3

18   Baio J, Wiggins L, Christensen DL, et al. Prevalence of autism spectrum disorder among children aged 8 years – autism and developmental disabilities monitoring network, 11 sites, United States, 2014. *MMWR Surveill Summ.* 2018;67(SS6):1–23. doi:10.15585/mmwr.ss6706a1

19   Li Q, Li Y, Liu B, et al. Prevalence of autism spectrum disorder among children and adolescents in the United States from 2019 to 2020. *JAMA Pediatr.* 2022;176(9):943–945. doi:10.1001/jamapediatrics.2022.1846

20   Evans B. How autism became autism: the radical transformation of a central concept of child development in Britain. *Hist Hum Sci.* 2013;26(3):3–31. doi:10.1177/0952695113484320

21   Howlin P. Adults with autism: changes in understanding since DSM-111. *J Autism Dev Disord.* 2021;51(12):4291–4308. doi:10.1007/s10803-020-04847-z

9. Personality and the Search for Normal

1   Dickson DH, Kelly IW. The 'Barnum effect' in personality assessment: a review of the literature. *Psychol Rep.* 1985;57(2):367–382. doi:10.2466/pr0.1985.57.2.367

2   McCrae RR, John OP. An introduction to the five-factor model and its applications. *J Pers.* 1992;60(2):175–215. doi:10.1111/j.1467-6494.1992.tb00970.x

3   Soldz S, Vaillant GE. The Big Five personality traits and the life course: a 45-year longitudinal study. *J Res Personal.* 1999;33(2):208–232. doi:10.1006/jrpe.1999.2243

4   Crocq MA. Milestones in the history of personality disorders. *Dialogues Clin Neurosci.* 2013;15(2):147–153. doi:10.31887/DCNS.2013.15.2/macrocq

5   Van Horn JD, Irimia A, Torgerson CM, Chambers MC, Kikinis R, Toga AW. Mapping connectivity damage in the case of Phineas Gage. *PLOS ONE.* 2012;7(5):e37454. doi:10.1371/journal.pone.0037454

6   Harlow JM. Recovery from the passage of an iron bar through the head. *Hist Psychiatry.* 1993;4(14):274–281. doi:10.1177/0957154X9300401407

7   Gouveia FV, Hamani C, Fonoff ET, et al. Amygdala and

hypothalamus: historical overview with focus on aggression. *Neurosurgery*. 2019;85(1):11. doi:10.1093/neuros/nyy635

8   Rajmohan V, Mohandas E. The limbic system. *Indian J Psychiatry*. 2007;49(2):132–139. doi:10.4103/0019-5545.33264

9   Blumer D. Evidence supporting the temporal lobe epilepsy personality syndrome. *Neurology*. 1999;53(5 Suppl 2):S9–12. https://pubmed.ncbi.nlm.nih.gov/10496229/

10   David AS, Fleminger S, Kopelman M, Lovestone S, Mellers J. *Lishman's Organic Psychiatry: A Textbook of Neuropsychiatry* Fourth Edition. Wiley-Blackwell, 2009, pp. 347–8.

11   Devinsky O, Najjar S. Evidence against the existence of a temporal lobe epilepsy personality syndrome. *Neurology*. 1999;53(5 Suppl 2):S13–25. doi:10.1111%2Fj.1535-7511.2007.00184.x

12   Report of the Royal Commission on the Care and Control of the Feebleminded. Great Britain Commissions for the Care and Control of the Feeble Minded, 1908, p. 324. https://archive.org/details/reportroyalcomm00mindgoog/page/n16/mode/2up

13   The ICD-10 classification of mental and behavioural disorders: clinical descriptions and diagnostic guidelines. World Health Organization, 1992. https://www.who.int/publications/i/item/9241544228

14   Jones DW. A history of borderline: disorder at the heart of psychiatry. *J Psychosoc Stud*. 2023;16(2):117–134. doi:10.1332/147867323X16871713092130

15   Pompili M, Girardi P, Ruberto A, Tatarelli R. Suicide in borderline personality disorder: a meta-analysis. *Nord J Psychiatry*. 2005;59(5):319–324. doi:10.1080/08039480500320025

16   Brodsky BS, Malone KM, Ellis SP, Dulit RA, Mann JJ. Characteristics of borderline personality disorder associated with suicidal behavior. *Am J Psychiatry*. 1997;154(12):1715–1719. doi:10.1176/AJP.154.12.1715

17   2024 ICD-10-CM Diagnosis Code F60.81: Narcissistic personality disorder. ICD10Data.com. Accessed 30 March 2024. https://www.icd10data.com/ICD10CM/Codes/F01-F99/F60-F69/F60-/F60.81

18   Atlas GD, Them MA. Narcissism and sensitivity to criticism: a preliminary investigation. *Curr Psychol*. 2008;27(1):62–76. doi:10.1007/S12144-008-9023-0/TABLES/5

19 Lee BX. 'Loser': a leading psychiatrist takes a detailed look into Trump's narcissistic pathologies. *Raw Story*. 11 August 2020. https://www.rawstory.com/2020/08/loser-a-leading-psychiatrist-takes-a-detailed-look-into-trumps-narcissistic-pathologies/?utm_source=push_notifications

20 Lilienfeld SO, Miller JD, Lynam DR. The Goldwater rule: perspectives from, and implications for, psychological science. *Perspect Psychol Sci*. 2018;13(1):3–27. doi:10.1177/1745691617727864

21 The Honourable Mr Justice MacDonald. *Kings College Hospital NHS Foundation Trust v C & Anor [2015] EWCOP 80*. 30 November 2015. http://www.bailii.org/ew/cases/EWCOP/2015/80.html

22 Pfohl B, Coryell W, Zimmerman M, Stangl D. DSM-III personality disorders: diagnostic overlap and internal consistency of individual DSM-III criteria. *Compr Psychiatry*. 1986;27(1):21–34. doi:10.1016/0010-440X(86)90066-0

23 ICD-11 for Mortality and Morbidity Statistics. Accessed 8 October 2024. https://icd.who.int/browse/2024-01/mms/en#37291724

24 ICD-11 for Mortality and Morbidity Statistics. Accessed 30 August 2024. https://icd.who.int/dev11/l-m/en#/http%3a%2f%2fid.who.int%2ficd%2fentity%2f37291724

25 Duggan C. Dangerous and severe personality disorder. *Br J Psychiatry*. 2011;198(6):431–433. doi:10.1192/bjp.bp.110.083048

26 Maden A. Dangerous and severe personality disorder: antecedents and origins. *British Journal of Psychiatry*. 2007;190(S49):s8–s11. doi:10.1192/bjp.190.5.s8

27 The offender personality disorder (OPD) pathway: a joint strategy for 2023 to 2028. NHS England. 1 December 2023. https://www.england.nhs.uk/long-read/the-offender-personality-disorder-pathway/

28 Lewis G, Appleby L. Personality disorder: the patients psychiatrists dislike. *Br J Psychiatry J Ment Sci*. 1988;153:44–49. doi:10.1192/bjp.153.1.44

10. Sex, Sexuality, Love and Gender

1 Drescher J. Out of DSM: Depathologizing homosexuality. *Behav Sci Basel Switz*. 2015;5(4):565–575. doi:10.3390/bs5040565

2   Smith G, Bartlett A, King M. Treatments of homosexuality in Britain since the 1950s – an oral history: the experience of patients. *BMJ*. 2004;328(7437):427. doi:10.1136/bmj.37984.442419.EE

3   King M, Bartlett A. British psychiatry and homosexuality. *Br J Psychiatry*. 1999;175(2):106–113. doi:10.1192/bjp.175.2.106

4   Silva D, Farias R, Cunha A, Peres R, Casagrande L. History and legacy of Alan Turing for computer science. *Int J Sci Res Manage*. 2024. doi:10.18535/ijsrm/v12i02.ec06

5   The origins of Section 28. The National Archives. Accessed 1 April 2024. https://beta.nationalarchives.gov.uk/explore-the-collection/stories/origins-section-28/

6   Sir James Anderton obituary. *Guardian*. 6 May 2022. https://www.theguardian.com/uk-news/2022/may/06/sir-james-anderton-obituary

7   Meerwijk EL, Sevelius JM. Transgender population size in the United States: a meta-regression of population-based probability samples. *Am J Public Health*. 2017;107(2):e1–e8. doi:10.2105/AJPH.2016.303578

8   Delahunt JW, Denison HJ, Sim DA, Bullock JJ, Krebs JD. Increasing rates of people identifying as transgender presenting to Endocrine Services in the Wellington region. *N Z Med J*. 2018;131(1468):33–42. https://pubmed.ncbi.nlm.nih.gov/29346355/

9   Gender identity, England and Wales. Office for National Statistics. Accessed 1 April 2024. https://www.ons.gov.uk/peoplepopulationandcommunity/culturalidentity/genderidentity/bulletins/genderidentityenglandandwales/census2021

10   Number of referrals to GIDS. Gender Identity Development Service. Accessed 6 September 2023. https://gids.nhs.uk/about-us/number-of-referrals/

11   Cass H. Gender medicine for children and young people is built on shaky foundations. Here is how we strengthen services. *BMJ*. 2024;385:q814. doi:10.1136/BMJ.Q814

12   Abbasi K. The Cass review: an opportunity to unite behind evidence informed care in gender medicine. *BMJ*. 2024;385:q837. doi:10.1136/BMJ.Q837

13   Transgender surgery isn't the solution. *WSJ*. 13 May 2016. https://www.wsj.com/articles/paul-mchugh-transgender-surgery-isnt-the-solution-1402615120

14   ICD-11 for Mortality and Morbidity Statistics. Accessed 9 October 2024. https://icd.who.int/browse/2024-01/mms/en#90875286

15   Hanna B, Desai R, Parekh T, Guirguis E, Kumar G, Sachdeva R. Psychiatric disorders in the U.S. transgender population. *Ann Epidemiol.* 2019;39:1–7.e1. doi:10.1016/j.annepidem.2019.09.009

16   Bockting WO, Miner MH, Swinburne Romine RE, Hamilton A, Coleman E. Stigma, mental health, and resilience in an online sample of the US transgender population. *Am J Public Health.* 2013;103(5):943–951. doi:10.2105/AJPH.2013.301241

17   Warrier V, Greenberg DM, Weir E, et al. Elevated rates of autism, other neurodevelopmental and psychiatric diagnoses, and autistic traits in transgender and gender-diverse individuals. *Nat Commun.* 2020;11(1):3959. doi:10.1038/s41467-020-17794-1

18   Erlangsen A, Jacobsen AL, Ranning A, Delamare AL, Nordentoft M, Frisch M. Transgender identity and suicide attempts and mortality in Denmark. *JAMA.* 2023;329(24):2145–2153. doi:10.1001/jama.2023.8627

19   Ruuska SM, Tuisku K, Holttinen T, Kaltiala R. All-cause and suicide mortalities among adolescents and young adults who contacted specialised gender identity services in Finland in 1996–2019: a register study. *BMJ Ment Health.* 2024;27(1). doi:10.1136/bmjment-2023-300940

11. Welcome to the Metaverse

1   Rigas A, Mainka T, Pringsheim T, et al. Distinguishing functional from primary tics: a study of expert video assessments. *J Neurol Neurosurg Psychiatry.* 2023;94(9):751–756. doi:10.1136/JNNP-2022-330822

2   Amorelli G, Martino D, Pringsheim T. Rapid onset functional tic-like disorder outbreak: a challenging differential diagnosis in the COVID-19 pandemic. *J Can Acad Child Adolesc Psychiatry.* 2022;31(3):144. https://www.ncbi.nlm.nih.gov/pmc/articles/PMC9275373/

3   Olvera C, Stebbins GT, Goetz CG, Kompoliti K. TikTok tics: a pandemic within a pandemic. *Mov Disord Clin Pract.* 2021;8(8):1200–1205. doi:10.1002/MDC3.13316

4   Heyman I, Liang H, Hedderly T. COVID-19 related increase in childhood tics and tic-like attacks. *Arch Dis Child.* 2021;106(5):420–421. doi:10.1136/archdischild-2021-321748

5   van Tulder M, Malmivaara A, Koes B. Repetitive strain injury.
         Lancet. 2007;369(9575):1815–1822. doi:10.1016/S0140-
         6736(07)60820-4

6   Harshbarger JL, Ahlers-Schmidt CR, Mayans L, Mayans D, Hawkins
         JH. Pro-anorexia websites: what a clinician should know. *Int J Eat
         Disord*. 2009;42(4):367–370. doi:10.1002/EAT.20608

7   Norris ML, Boydell KM, Pinhas L, Katzman DK. Ana and the
         internet: a review of pro-anorexia websites. *Int J Eat Disord*.
         2006;39(6):443–447. doi:10.1002/EAT.20305

8   Harris EC, Barraclough B. Excess mortality of mental disorder. *Br J
         Psychiatry J Ment Sci*. 1998 Jul;173:11–53. doi:10.1192/BJP.173.1.11

9   Bardone-Cone AM, Cass KM. What does viewing a pro-anorexia
         website do? An experimental examination of website exposure
         and moderating effects. *Int J Eat Disord*. 2007;40(6):537–548.
         doi:10.1002/EAT.20396

10   Jett S, La Porte DJ, Wanchisn J. Impact of exposure to pro-eating
         disorder websites on eating behaviour in college women. *Eur Eat
         Disord Rev*. 2010;18(5):410–416. doi:10.1002/ERV.1009

11   Mento C, Silvestri MC, Muscatello MRA, et al. Psychological
         impact of pro-anorexia and pro-eating disorder websites on
         adolescent females: a systematic review. *Int J Environ Res Public
         Health*. 2021;18(4):1–14. doi:10.3390/IJERPH18042186

12   Madigan S, Racine N, Vaillancourt T, et al. Changes in depression
         and anxiety among children and adolescents from before to
         during the COVID-19 pandemic: a systematic review and
         meta-analysis. *JAMA Pediatr*. 2023;177(6):567–581. doi:10.1001/
         jamapediatrics.2023.0846

13   Racine N, McArthur BA, Cooke JE, Eirich R, Zhu J, Madigan S.
         Global prevalence of depressive and anxiety symptoms in children
         and adolescents during COVID-19: a meta-analysis. *JAMA Pediatr*.
         2021;175(11):1142–1150. doi:10.1001/jamapediatrics.2021.2482

14   Waller J. A forgotten plague: making sense of dancing mania. *Lancet*.
         2009;373(9664):624–625. doi:10.1016/S0140-6736(09)60386-X

15   Man dies after 3-day Internet gaming binge. CNN. 19 January
         2015. https://edition.cnn.com/2015/01/19/world/taiwan-gamer-
         death/index.html

16   Kuperczko D, Kenyeres P, Darnai G, Kovacs N, Janszky J. Sudden
         gamer death: non-violent death cases linked to playing video games.
         BMC Psychiatry. 2022;22(1). doi:10.1186/S12888-022-04373-5

17   Feng W, Ramo DE, Chan SR, Bourgeois JA. Internet gaming disorder: trends in prevalence 1998–2016. *Addict Behav.* 2017;75:17–24. doi:10.1016/J.ADDBEH.2017.06.010

18   Przybylski AK, Weinstein N, Murayama K. Internet gaming disorder: investigating the clinical relevance of a new phenomenon. *Am J Psychiatry.* 2017;174(3):230–235. doi:10.1176/APPI.AJP.2016.16020224

19   Aarseth E, Bean AM, Boonen H, et al. Scholars' open debate paper on the World Health Organization ICD-11 Gaming Disorder proposal. *J Behav Addict.* 2017;6(3):267–270. doi:10.1556/2006.5.2016.088

20   Zastrow M. Is video game addiction really an addiction? *Proc Natl Acad Sci U S A.* 2017;114(17):4268–4272. https://doi.org/10.1073/pnas.1705077114

21   Clark L. Disordered gambling: the evolving concept of behavioral addiction. *Ann NY Acad Sci.* 2014;1327(1):46–61. doi:10.1111/nyas.12558

22   ICD-11 for Mortality and Morbidity Statistics. Accessed 9 October 2024. https://icd.who.int/browse/2024-01/mms/en#1630268048

23   Kwon M, Lee JY, Won WY, et al. Development and validation of a smartphone addiction scale (SAS). *PLOS ONE.* 2013;8(2). doi:10.1371/journal.pone.0056936

24   Sohn SY, Krasnoff L, Rees P, Kalk NJ, Carter B. The association between smartphone addiction and sleep: a UK cross-sectional study of young adults. *Front Psychiatry.* 2021;12:629407. doi:10.3389/FPSYT.2021.629407/BIBTEX

25   Olson JA, Sandra DA, Colucci ÉS, et al. Smartphone addiction is increasing across the world: A meta-analysis of 24 countries. *Comput Hum Behav.* 2022;129:107138. doi:10.1016/J.CHB.2021.107138

26   Panova T, Carbonell X. Is smartphone addiction really an addiction? *J Behav Addict.* 2018;7(2):252–259. doi:10.1556/2006.7.2018.49

27   Campagna JDA, Bowsher B. Prevalence of body dysmorphic disorder and muscle dysmorphia among entry-level military personnel. *Mil Med.* 2016;181(5):494–501. doi:10.7205/MILMED-D-15-00118

28   Pope Jr HG, Olivardia R, Gruber A, Borowiecki J. Evolving ideals of male body image as seen through action toys. *Int J Eat*

Disord. 1999;26(1):65–72. doi:https://doi.org/10.1002/(sici)1098-108x(199907)26:1<65::aid-eat8>3.0.co;2-d

29   Donini LM, Marsili D, Graziani MP, Imbriale M, Cannella C. Orthorexia nervosa: a preliminary study with a proposal for diagnosis and an attempt to measure the dimension of the phenomenon. *Eat Weight Disord.* 2004;9(2):151–157. doi:10.1007/BF03325060/METRICS

30   Vuorre M, Przybylski AK. Global well-being and mental health in the internet age. *Clin Psychol Sci.* 2023;12(5). https://doi.org/10.1177/21677026231207791

12. Risk

1   Chan MKY, Bhatti H, Meader N, et al. Predicting suicide following self-harm: systematic review of risk factors and risk scales. *Br J Psychiatry.* 2016;209(4):277–283. doi:10.1192/bjp.bp.115.170050

2   Large MM, Ryan CJ, Carter G, Kapur N. Can we usefully stratify patients according to suicide risk? *BMJ.* 2017;359. doi:10.1136/bmj.j4627

3   Wu CY, Chang CK, Hayes RD, Broadbent M, Hotopf M, Stewart R. Clinical risk assessment rating and all-cause mortality in secondary mental healthcare: the South London and Maudsley NHS Foundation Trust Biomedical Research Centre (SLAM BRC) Case Register. *Psychol Med.* 2012;42(8):1581–1590. doi:10.1017/S0033291711002698

4   Census 2021: workforce figures for consultant psychiatrists, specialty doctor psychiatrists and physician associates in mental health. The Royal College of Psychiatrists. Accessed 14 October 2024. https://www.rcpsych.ac.uk/docs/default-source/improving-care/workforce/census-2021-completed-draft.pdf?sfvrsn=191319cb_2

5   Homicide in England and Wales: year ending March 2023. Office for National Statistics. Accessed 18 October 2024. https://www.ons.gov.uk/peoplepopulationandcommunity/crimeandjustice/articles/homicideinenglandandwales/yearendingmarch2023#circumstances-and-location-of-homicides

6   Steinkamp J, Kantrowitz JJ, Airan-Javia S. Prevalence and sources of duplicate information in the electronic medical record. *JAMA Netw Open.* 2022;5(9):e2233348-e2233348. doi:10.1001/jamanetworkopen.2022.33348

7   Hardwick P. Formarrhoea. *Psychiatr Bull.* 2003;27(10):388–389. doi:10.1192/pb.27.10.388

8   Tyrer P. Has the closure of psychiatric beds gone too far? Yes. *BMJ.* 2011;343. doi:10.1136/bmj.d7457

9   Number of NHS mental health beds down by 25% since 2010, analysis shows. *Guardian.* 5 July 2021. https://www.theguardian. com/society/2021/jul/05/number-of-nhs-mental-health-beds-down-by-25-since-2010-analysis-shows

10   Exploring mental health inpatient capacity across sustainability and transformation partnerships in England. Strategy Unit, NHS Midlands and Lancashire. November 2019. https://www. strategyunitwm.nhs.uk/sites/default/files/2019-11/Exploring%20 Mental%20Health%20Inpatient%20Capacity%20accross%20 Sustainability%20and%20Transformation%20Partnerships%20in%20 England%20-%20191030_1.pdf

11   Service capacity in England. Royal College of Psychiatrists. Accessed 3 April 2022. https://www.rcpsych.ac.uk/improving-care/campaigning-for-better-mental-health-policy/service-capacity-in-england

12   Casey P, Dunn G, Kelly BD, et al. The prevalence of suicidal ideation in the general population: results from the Outcome of Depression International Network (ODIN) study. *Soc Psychiatry Psychiatr Epidemiol.* 2008;43(4):299–304. doi:10.1007/s00127-008-0313-5

13   Ivey-Stephenson AZ, Crosby AE, Hoenig JM, Gyawali S, Park-Lee E, Hedden, SL. Suicidal thoughts and behaviors among adults aged ≥ 18 years – United States, 2015–2019. *MMWR Surveill Summ.* 2022;71:1–19. https://doi.org/10.15585/mmwr.ss7101a1

13. Tomorrow's World

1   Voice J, Ponterio JM, Lakhi N. Psychosis secondary to an incidental teratoma: a 'heads-up' for psychiatrists and gynecologists. *Arch Womens Ment Health.* 2017;20(5):703–707. doi:10.1007/S00737-017-0751-8/FIGURES/1

2   Benros ME, Pedersen MG, Rasmussen H, Eaton WW, Nordentoft M, Mortensen PB. A nationwide study on the risk of autoimmune diseases in individuals with a personal or a family history of schizophrenia and related psychosis. *Am J Psychiatry.* 2014;171(2):218–226. doi:10.1176/appi.ajp.2013.13010086

3   Dassa D, Azorin JM, Ledoray V, Sambuc R, Giudicelli S. Season of birth and schizophrenia: sex difference. *Prog Neuropsychopharmacol Biol Psychiatry*. 1996;20(2):243–251. doi:10.1016/0278-5846(95)00307-X

4   Ripke S, Neale BM, Corvin A, et al. Biological insights from 108 schizophrenia-associated genetic loci. *Nature*. 2014 5117510. 2014;511(7510):421–427. doi:10.1038/nature13595

5   Schmack K, Bosc M, Ott T, Sturgill JF, Kepecs A. Striatal dopamine mediates hallucination-like perception in mice. *Science*. 2021;372(6537):eabf4740. doi:10.1126/science.abf4740

6   Kotov R, Jonas KG, Carpenter WT, et al. Validity and utility of Hierarchical Taxonomy of Psychopathology (HiTOP): I. Psychosis superspectrum. *World Psychiatry*. 2020;19(2):151–172. doi:10.1002/wps.20730

7   Kendler KS. The nature of psychiatric disorders. *World Psychiatry*. 2016;15(1):5–12. doi:10.1002/wps.20292

8   Blashfield RK, Keeley JW, Flanagan EH, Miles SR. The cycle of classification: DSM-I through DSM-5. *Annu Rev Clin Psychol*. 2014;10:25–51. https://doi.org/10.1146/annurev-clinpsy-032813-153639

9   Controversy over DSM-5: new mental health guide. *Nursing Times*. 24 August 2013. https://www.nursingtimes.net/news/behind-the-headlines/controversy-over-dsm-5-new-mental-health-guide-24-08-2013/

10   DSM-5 is a guide, not a bible – simply ignore its 10 worst changes. *Psychiatric Times*. 5 December 2012. https://www.psychiatrictimes.com/view/dsm-5-guide-not-biblesimply-ignore-its-10-worst-changes

11   Families and households in the UK: 2023. Office for National Statistics. Accessed 9 August 2024. https://www.ons.gov.uk/peoplepopulationandcommunity/birthsdeathsandmarriages/families/bulletins/familiesandhouseholds/2023

12   Putnam RD. Bowling alone: America's declining social capital. *J Democr*. 1995;6(1):65–78.

13   Mushtaq R, Shoib S, Shah T, Mushtaq S. Relationship between loneliness, psychiatric disorders and physical health? A review on the psychological aspects of loneliness. *J Clin Diagn Res*. 2014;8(9):WE01–WE04. doi:10.7860/JCDR/2014/10077.4828

14   Sudimac S, Sale V, Kühn S. How nature nurtures: amygdala activity
          decreases as the result of a one-hour walk in nature. *Mol Psychiatry*.
          2022;27(11):4446–4452. doi:10.1038/s41380-022-01720-6

14. Epilogue

1   Zachar P, First MB, Kendler KS. The bereavement exclusion
          debate in the DSM-5: a history. 2017;5(5):890–906.
          doi:10.1177/2167702617711284
2   Frances A: My biggest DSM-IV regret: our broadening the autism
          definition that has led to such massive, careless over-diagnosis.
          27 April 2023. https://x.com/AllenFrancesMD/status/1651413305
          662251008?lang=en-GB
3   Grief vs depression – one last word. *Psychology Today*. 30 April
          2010. https://www.psychologytoday.com/intl/blog/dsm5-in-
          distress/201004/grief-vs-depression-one-last-word
4   Kleinman A. Culture, bereavement, and psychiatry. *Lancet*.
          2012:379(9816);608–609. doi:10.1016/S0140-6736(12)60258-X
5   Thieleman K, Cacciatore J, Frances A. Rates of prolonged grief
          disorder: considering relationship to the person who died and
          cause of death. *J Affect Disord*. 2023;339:832–837. doi:10.1016/J.
          JAD.2023.07.094

Index

acetylcholine, 59
adjustment disorders, 230
ageing, fear of, 53
aggression, 135, 143
Alzheimer's disease, 52, 57, 59
American Journal of Psychiatry, 123, 191, 217
amnesia, 48–9
amphetamines, 121
amygdala, 143
anaesthesia, 13, 22
anal retentives, 159
anankastia, 158
angina, 22
animal magnetism, 116
anorexia, 175, 184–6
antibiotics, 11, 38
antidepressants, 8, 13, 22–3, 25, 32, 84, 88, 91–6, 101, 126, 229, 231
antipsychiatry, 9, 15, 24–5
anxiety, 9, 42, 97, 109, 152, 169, 186, 188, 194, 216, 230
  and ADHD, 119, 122, 127, 129
  and autism, 133–4, 136–7
  as cultural category, 35
  and depression, 86, 90
  diagnosis, 224–6
  and gender identity, 173, 176
  and memory, 52–5

and PMDD, 31–2
and risk, 206
and trigger warnings, 112
appetite, 31, 84, 93, 96
asbestosis, 182
Asperger's syndrome, 135–6
Astra-Zeneca, 42
asylums, 8, 12–15
attention deficit hyperactivity disorder (ADHD), 8, 119–33
  'masked symptoms', 129
  and pharmaceutical industry, 130–2
autism, 4, 35, 130, 133–7, 231
  and gender identity, 175–6
autism spectrum disorder (ASD), 3–4, 134, 136–7
aversion therapy, 166
awareness raising campaigns, 36, 120, 129

Barnum effect, 140
behavioural conditioning, 165
behavioural contracts, 148–9
bereavement, 2, 82, 230–3
beta blockers, 22–3
bipolar disorder, 9–10, 24,

96, 98, 129–30
blood pressure, 147, 158, 190
Boer War, 104
Borsboom, Denny, 30, 34
bowling, 226
brain scans, 28, 49, 53, 58–9, 77, 160
brain tumours, 143
Bratton, Doug, 117
breast cancer, 156, 201
breathlessness, 39
British Journal of Psychiatry, 71, 211
British Medical Journal, 3, 57, 172
bulimia, 185
Burns, Robert, 139

Cahalan, Susannah, 19
cardiology, 227
Cass report, 171–2
catatonia, 21, 83
Charcot, Jean-Martin, 102
childhood abuse, 47–8, 217
chlorpromazine, 13
cholera, 182
cholinesterase inhibitors, 59
Choosing Wisely campaign, 93
Cochrane Database of Systematic Reviews, 97, 105–6
computational psychiatry, 218–22

260